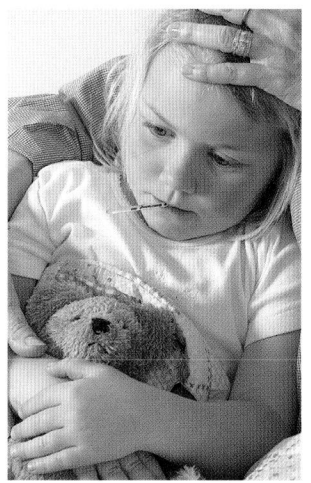

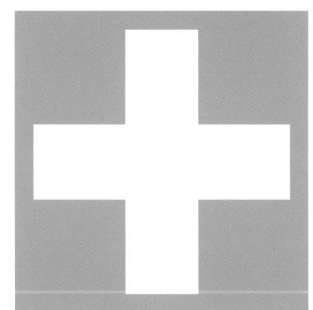

FIRST
AID
for Family
Emergencies

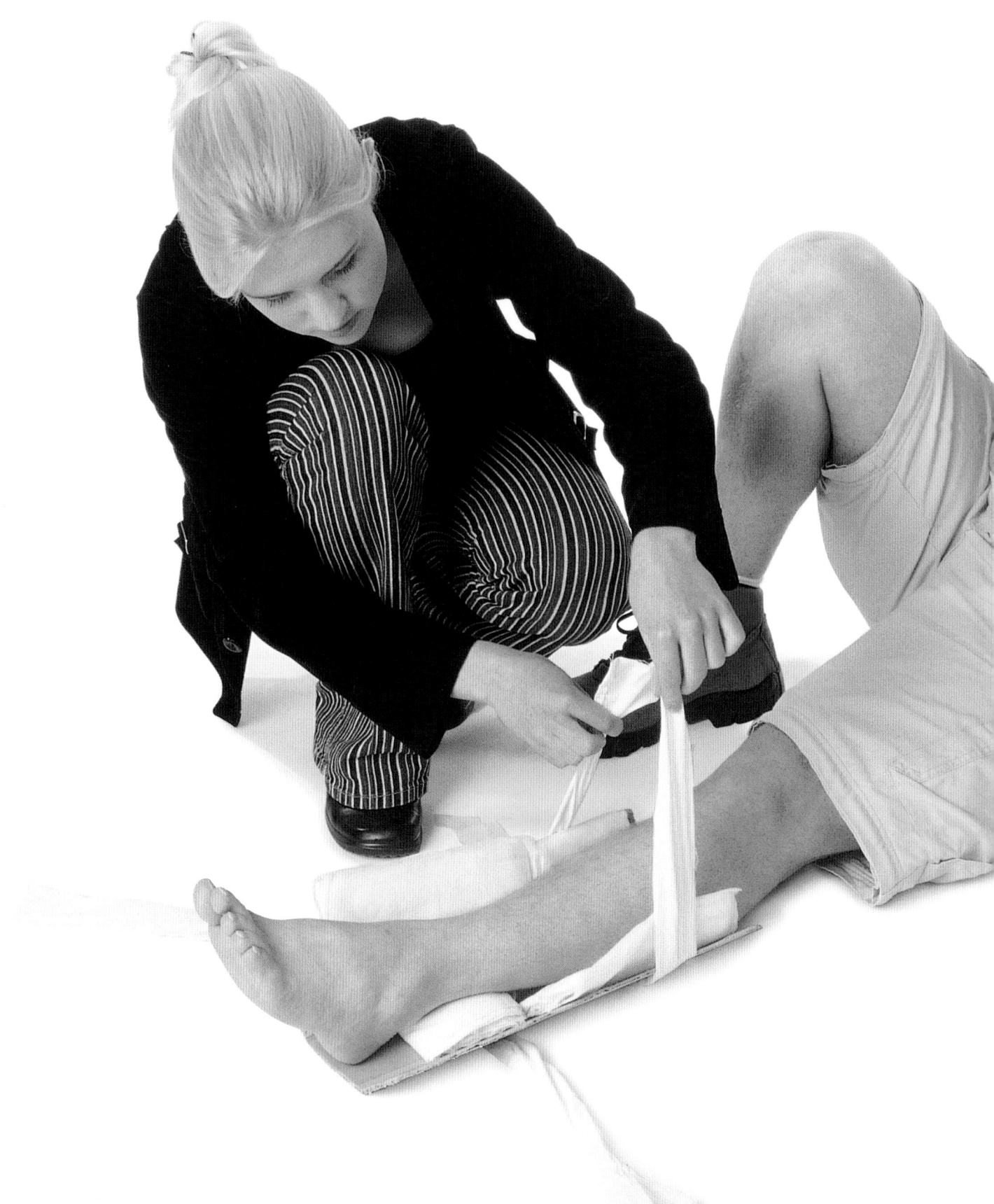

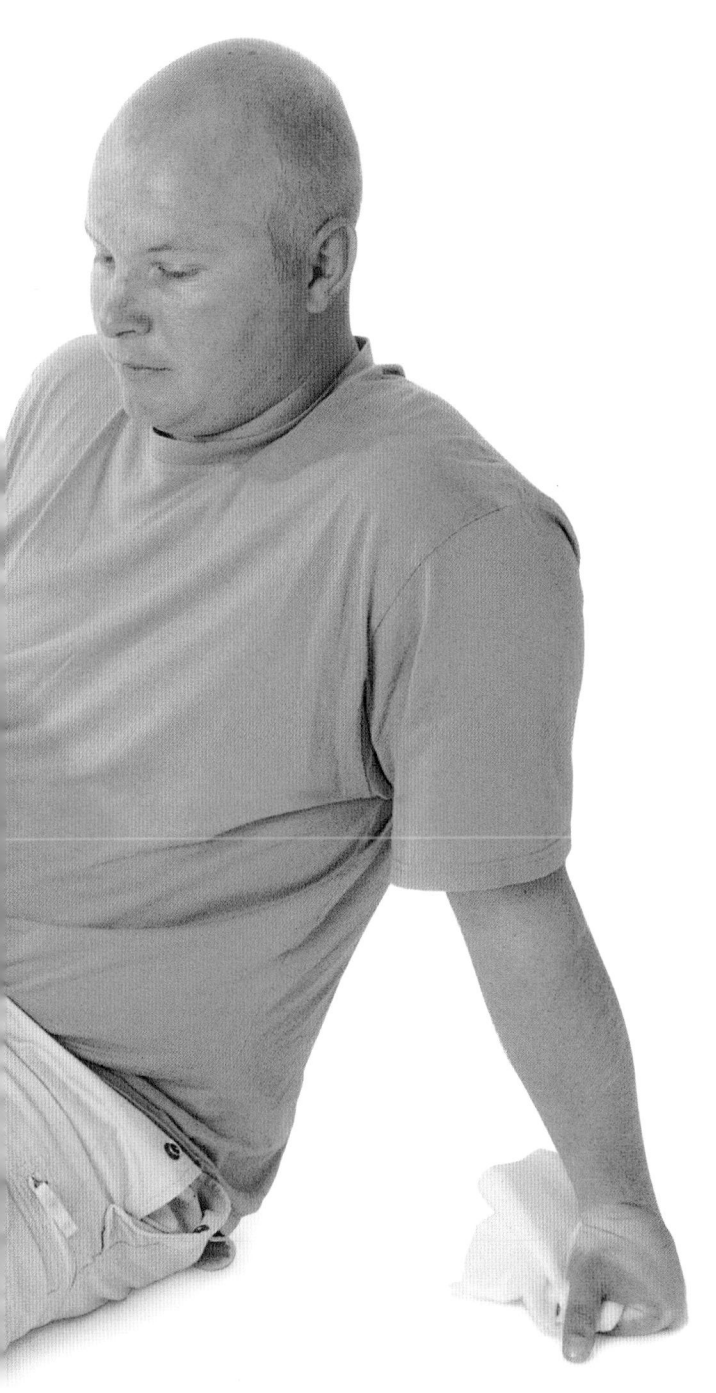

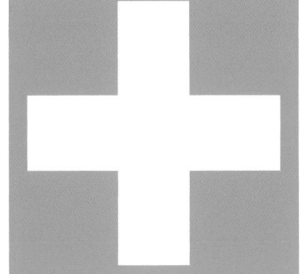

FIRST
AID
for Family
Emergencies

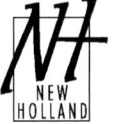

NEW
HOLLAND

Rod Baker and Dr David Bass

First published in 2005 by New Holland Publishers
London • Cape Town • Sydney • Auckland
www.newhollandpublishers.com

Garfield House
86 Edgware Rd
London W2 2EA
United Kingdom

80 McKenzie St
Cape Town
8001
South Africa

14 Aquatic Drive
Frenchs Forest
NSW 2086
Australia

218 Lake Rd
Northcote
Auckland
New Zealand

Commissioning editor: *Alfred LeMaitre*
Editor: *Gill Gordon*
Designer: *Richard MacArthur*
Illustrators: *Ian Lusted, Stephen Felmore*
Picture research: *Karla Kik, Tamlyn McGeean*

Production: *Myrna Collins*
Proofreaders/indexers: *Elizabeth Wilson,*
Sylvia Grobbelaar
Consultants: *Dr Malcolm Henry;*
Sarah Colles (Home Safety Adviser, RoSPA);

ISBN 1 84330 860 6 (hb)
ISBN 1 84357 082 1 (pb)

Reproduction by Resolution Colour (Pty) Ltd., Cape Town, South Africa
Printed and bound in the UK by Butler and Tanner

1 3 5 7 9 10 8 6 4 2

The advice contained in this book is intended for reference only and cannot replace the advice of a qualified physician.
A licensed physician should be consulted for the diagnosis and treatment of any and all medical conditions and
emergencies. The publisher assumes no liability for any consequences, loss, injury or inconvenience sustained
by any person using this book or the advice given in it.

CONTENTS

HOME CARE

SAFETY AROUND THE HOME

SAFETY OUTDOORS

WATER SAFETY

APPENDIX

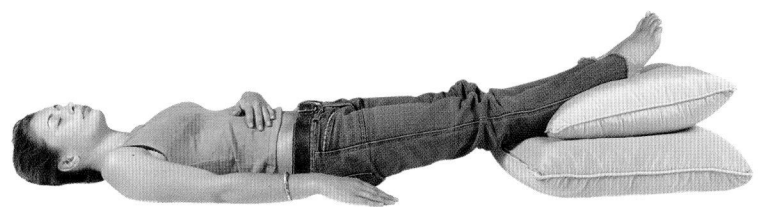

FIRST STEPS
TO TAKE

We all hope that we will never have to experience and be called upon to assist in a situation requiring first aid, but by preparing yourself beforehand you will know what to do.

A knowledge of basic first aid procedures will help you to remain calm and efficient. It will help you to know what to do and – equally importantly – you will know what not to do. It will also enable you to improvise, using whatever items are available to achieve a favourable result.

The individual medical emergencies in this book provide a range of specific do-and-don't instructions but be sure to learn the basics at least. By attending a recognized first aid course you could end up doing someone else a greater favour – like saving their life!

IN THIS SECTION

Coping in an emergency

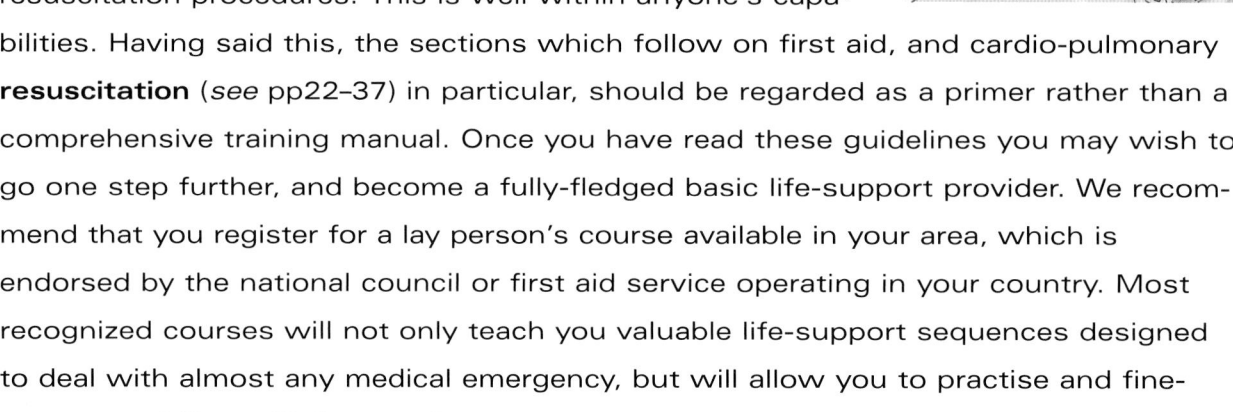

In an emergency situation, the desire to provide meaningful care and comfort can easily dissolve into blind panic unless you have certain basic skills and a systematic approach to resuscitation procedures. This is well within anyone's capabilities. Having said this, the sections which follow on first aid, and cardio-pulmonary **resuscitation** (*see* pp22–37) in particular, should be regarded as a primer rather than a comprehensive training manual. Once you have read these guidelines you may wish to go one step further, and become a fully-fledged basic life-support provider. We recommend that you register for a lay person's course available in your area, which is endorsed by the national council or first aid service operating in your country. Most recognized courses will not only teach you valuable life-support sequences designed to deal with almost any medical emergency, but will allow you to practise and fine-tune your skills on lifelike manikins.

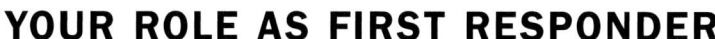

YOUR ROLE AS FIRST RESPONDER

Most injuries and serious medical emergencies occur without warning in places or situations that may be a considerable distance away from a hospital, doctor's surgery or ambulance station. Although ambulance personnel, fire-fighters and lifeguards are extensively trained to deal with emergency situations they may not be able to get to the scene of an accident on time. The outcome, and sometimes the difference between life and death, often depends on just two factors:

· the speed with which basic life support measures can be provided
· whether there is one adult on the scene who can calmly assess the nature and severity of the situation, call for the appropriate assistance, and, if necessary, commence **resuscitation procedures** (*see* pp22–37) while waiting for help to arrive.

Particularly in life-threatening situations such as **near-drowning** (*see* p21 and p163), **choking** (*see* p34)

and severe bleeding from a deep **laceration** (*see* pp84–5), a casualty's survival may depend upon whether the first person on the scene, i.e. the first responder, can initiate effective resuscitation while waiting for professional help to arrive.

As a parent or grandparent, teacher, childminder, sports coach or simply a concerned individual who wants to be able to 'make a difference', you may wish to gain the skills necessary to act as the first responder in a range of medical emergencies. If you do, the step-by-step guidelines, tips and precautions contained in this book should help you to act systematically and usefully in those precious early minutes after serious illness or injury strike.

In simple terms, first aid includes a wide range of guidelines and skills that enable you to provide effective assistance to someone who is ill or injured, and to do so quickly, regardless of the location, and with a bare minimum of medical equipment.

Whatever the nature of the emergency, the basic principles of first aid remain the same:

- Call an ambulance earlier rather than later
- Carefully assess the situation
- Protect yourself AND the casualty from unnecessary danger
- Begin first aid as the casualty requires
- Continue first aid until the casualty recovers, or until help arrives

Calling for help

In many instances, a first responder is able to assist quickly and efficiently. There are situations, however, where the exact nature and severity of the problem may not be clearly apparent. Call for assistance before commencing first aid if the casualty is:

- unconscious, drowsy, or disorientated
- having difficulty breathing or is not breathing at all
- suffering from multiple injuries, burns or electrical injuries
- bleeding heavily from one or more wounds
- a victim of poisoning

In any situation where you are unsure as to the cause of collapse or injury, another reliable adult should be instructed to telephone for assistance while you commence first aid. If no one is available to do this, telephone for help yourself before starting resuscitation.

Who you should call will depend on the emergency services in the area where you live. Whether that happens to be an ambulance service, fire brigade, hospital emergency room or a private doctor, always ensure that the telephone numbers are written down next to your home telephone and in your diary, and included in the directory of your mobile phone.

Assessing the situation

Being an effective first responder calls for a balance between enthusiasm and good judgement. In other words: look before you leap, regardless of the severity of the emergency. If you are alone, for example, and faced with more than one casualty, you may need to assess them all and decide who requires your assistance most urgently. Each situation you encounter as a first provider should be calmly and objectively assessed before you decide exactly how to handle it most effectively.

Protect yourself and the casualty from unnecessary danger

If you need to provide first aid in a potentially dangerous situation, good judgement is essential to ensure everyone's safety, including your own. Even if you are the only one able to provide help you must never put your own life at risk to save another.

Giving first aid

Even if the cause of a collapse (*see* p21) is unknown, commencing resuscitation without delay remains a priority. When a casualty is unconscious, in shock, or is having difficulty breathing, the speed with which you establish this and set about restoring normal breathing and blood circulation is the single most important factor. Your quick response will give the casualty the best possible chance of recovery.

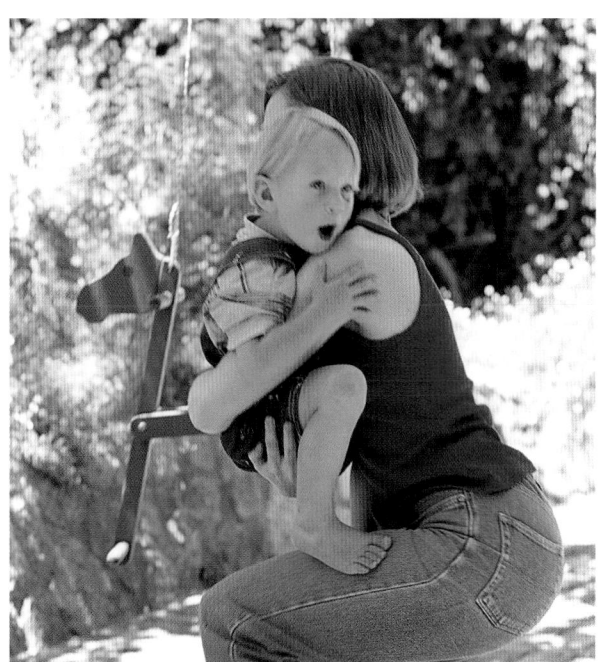

If you have an emergency in your home, call on a friend or neighbour to take care of small children so that you can deal with it.

CALLING FOR HELP

In many instances, the emergency care required from you as a first aid provider may be fairly straightforward, and no outside help may be necessary. At other times, however, the extent or severity of the problem may not be clearly apparent, particularly in someone who is unconscious or has collapsed for no apparent reason. Note the distinction between asking a bystander for help and calling the emergency services, referred to in this book as 'Call an ambulance'.

Having assessed the casualty, call for assistance in the following situations:

- A casualty who is having difficulty breathing or is not breathing at all
- A casualty with multiple injuries, head or back injuries, or extensive burns
- A casualty who is bleeding heavily from one or more wounds
- A casualty who is unconscious, feeling disoriented or drowsy
- Suspected poisoning
- Any situation where you are unsure as to the cause of the casualty's collapse or injury
- Any incident involving more than one badly injured casualty

Ideally, you should instruct a second, reliable adult to telephone for assistance while you commence basic life support (*see* **resuscitation** pp22–37). If no one is available to do this, call an ambulance yourself, before commencing **rescue breaths** (*see* p26).

Whom to call for help will depend on what services are available in the area where you live (or where the accident or incident took place). Be it an ambulance, paramedic, the local police, a hospital emergency room or the number of a private doctor, ensure that emergency numbers are written down clearly and always kept next to your home telephone, as well as in your diary and in the directory of your mobile phone. (*See* p175 for an **emergency list**.) Don't neglect to inform your children – even toddlers are able to memorize their home address and the (usually simple) numbers to dial for emergency response.

What to say on the phone

When you call an emergency service provider, you must be able to provide some basic information. Speak clearly, so that you don't have to repeat yourself and lose time:

- **Your name and telephone number** (fixed or mobile) you are calling from.
- A **brief description** of what has happened (e.g. 'a man has collapsed and he isn't breathing').
- Your **location**; a physical address is needed, and possibly directions as well.

Do not hang up the telephone until you are told to do so. The dispatcher may be able to give you information that will assist you with the casualty, or they may require you to provide additional information for the medics.

EMERGENCY CONTACTS

Ambulance/emergency service ....

Hospital ....

Doctor ....

Fire brigade ....

Police ....

Poison centre ....

Relative ....

Neighbour ....

School ....

Work ....

Pharmacy ....

Dentist ....

Vet ....

Electricity ....

Gas ....

Water ....

Insurance company ....

PERSONAL SAFETY AND INFECTION CONTROL

When you encounter an injured person, particularly someone who is not known to you, you should aim to protect yourself and the casualty against the risk of infectious disease before commencing resuscitation or providing first aid treatment. Although the risk of becoming infected with the Human Immunodeficiency Virus (HIV) is widely known and justly feared, first aid providers are at risk of infection by other viruses, such as Hepatitis B, if they come into contact with contaminated blood or body fluids of an infected person. To reduce the risk of infection, we strongly recommend that you make a habit of employing a basic minimum of infection control measures – commonly referred to as 'standard precautions' – when putting your first aid skills into practice, whether for the benefit of your own family, or a complete stranger.

PROTECT YOURSELF

Once you have completed a recognized basic first-aid course and are ready to volunteer your skills in a medical emergency, you should carry a few pairs of surgical gloves and a sealed, disposable resuscitation face shield around with you just in case. The gloves need not necessarily be sterile, just clean and unbroken. The face shield has a one-way valve which prevents saliva or blood passing from the casualty's mouth into yours. Neither of these items takes up much room, and can easily be carried in a bag or jacket pocket. Standard precautions are especially important if:

· There is a risk of coming into contact with blood or other body fluids, for example when performing mouth-to-mouth resuscitation, or if the person is bleeding from any site.
· You have a fresh skin wound or skin rash on your own hands or face.

· You live in a country or region where there is a high prevalence of infectious hepatitis or Human Immunodeficiency Virus (HIV).

If you must give life support without surgical gloves, even if it appears that no contamination with body fluids has occurred, always wash your hands and face with soap and water immediately afterwards. If you are at all worried abut the possibility of having contracted any form of infection during resuscitation, consult your doctor.

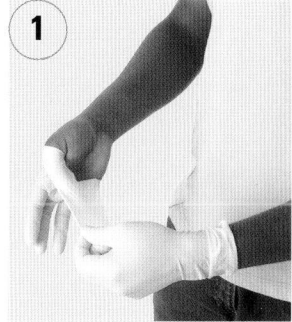 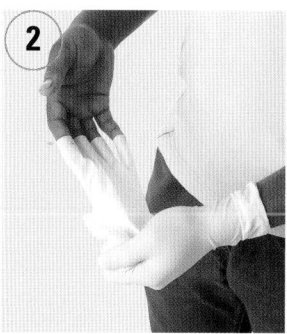

1. *Remove the glove from one hand, turning it inside out as you do so.*

2. *Ensure that no part of the used glove touches any part of your skin.*

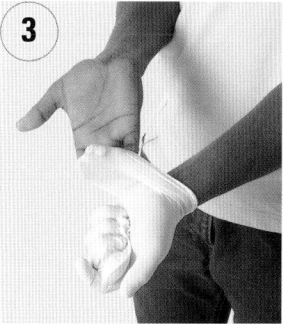 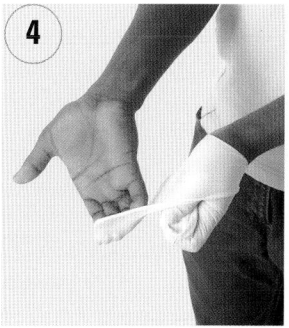

3. *Holding the used glove in your gloved hand, slip your fingers inside the second glove.*

4. *Remove the second glove by turning it inside out to enclose all the contaminated surfaces.*

First-aid kits

You should always have first-aid kit handy in your home and vehicle, and whenever you engage in outdoor pursuits such as hiking or camping. Many commercially available ready-made kits suit the most basic of needs, but consider making up your own kit or supplementing a bought one, so that it takes into account the ages and specific requirements of your family members. Keep a first-aid manual or instruction booklet in the kit and ensure that all medicines are clearly labelled as to their particular usage and dosage. It is a good idea to check on expiry dates from time to time to ensure that your supply is not out of date. Tape an accurate list of emergency numbers (preferably laminated) to the inside of the lid. First-aid kits and their contents should be safe from small, enquiring hands.

TIPS

- Keep the first-aid kit in one place so that everyone in the family knows where to find it.
- Humidity and steam accelerate deterioration of medications. Store the kit in a cool, dry place such as a locked bedroom cupboard.
- Check the contents regularly. Replace items that have expired. Be familiar with the contents and know exactly how to use it.
- Foil packs last longer than loose pills.
- Retain the original packaging of tablets complete with inserts.
- Most medication is dispensed in the correct quantity to treat a condition and prescribed courses must be followed as directed. Dispose of leftover medication or return it to your pharmacist.
- Never keep unidentified medication.

GENERAL PURPOSE ITEMS

- Pack of disposable surgical gloves
- Protective face shield for resuscitation
- Antiseptic liquid, centrimide solution (1%) or individually wrapped antiseptic wipes for cleaning wounds
- All-purpose antiseptic cream or ointment
- Blunt-nosed scissors
- Cotton wool and cotton-tipped swabs/buds
- Paper tissues
- Eye drops/saline eye solution and an eye bath
- Dosage spoon or medicine dropper
- Thermometer and/or heat-sensitive strip
- Tweezers and new pins or sewing needles (useful for prising out splinters)
- Petroleum jelly or aqueous cream
- Antihistamine cream or lotion to stop itches

BANDAGES AND DRESSINGS

- Waterproof and fabric adhesive plasters in a range of different shapes and sizes, including butterfly bandages to close wounds
- Rolls of adhesive bandage (fabric and waterproof) in 75mm and 100mm widths

- Gauze bandages (75mm and 100mm)
- Sterile gauze dressings or pads
- Packaged burn dressings
- Tubular bandage for treating finger wounds
- Elasticized bandages or strappings
- Two or three triangular bandages
- Sterile eye dressings
- Safety pins or bandage clips

MEDICATIONS TO KEEP AT HOME

Choice of medications will depend on who lives in your home. If you have small children, keep adult and paediatric medication and give dosages strictly in accordance with recommended guidelines.
- Aspirin or paracetamol tablets or capsules
- Antacid tablets, liquid or powders

- Anti-diarrhoea tablets (not advised for children)
- Cough syrup and throat lozenges
- Anti-inflammatory tablets and/or cream

USEFUL ITEMS TO KEEP IN THE CAR

- Large, clean plastic bag or bin liner (to use as a ground cover in an emergency)
- Waterless hand-cleaner or 'wet wipes'
- Paper tissues or toilet paper
- Old towel or blanket, or a space blanket
- Torch with separate (unused) batteries, or one that plugs into the vehicle's cigarette lighter
- Empty container for water. (When setting out on a long journey, carry fresh water.) If you carry fuel, ensure that all containers are clearly marked

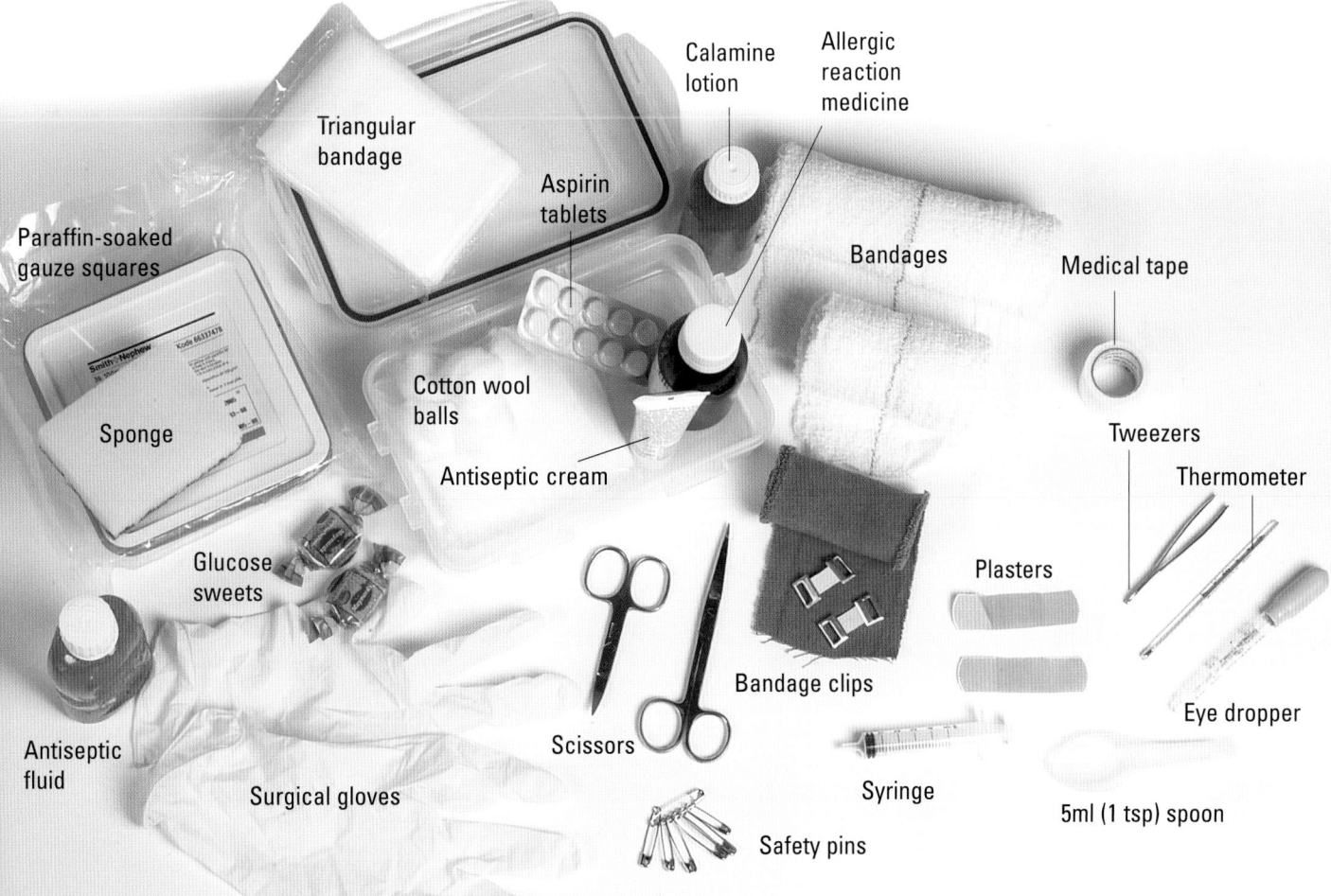

Be familiar with the contents of your first-aid kit and know how to use it.

Accidents

If you are the first person at the scene of an accident involving serious injury you need to be able to take charge and direct additional helpers until qualified medical support arrives. To do this effectively, you must remain calm and concentrate on what you have to do. The sooner effective treatment starts, the better the potential outcome. The worst situation is when breathing ceases or the heart stops beating. These take precedence over anything else. If you are at the scene of an accident involving multiple casualties, first attention must be on those who are not breathing, no matter how bad other injuries may seem. Time is critical, so remain focused and follow the guidelines given here. Details of the **rescue breathing procedure** can be found on pages 22–37.

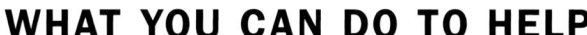

WHAT YOU CAN DO TO HELP

Determine priorities
- As soon as possible, check the casualty's **airway and breathing** (*see* p22). If there is more than one casualty, check them all and open the airway of anyone whose breathing has stopped or is failing.
- Place unconscious, but breathing casualties in the **recovery position** (*see* p25).
- Check if there is any uncontrolled bleeding. Get either the casualty or a bystander to help control the bleeding by putting pressure on the wound.
- Serious accidents often produce more than one injury. Once breathing and circulation are established, check for other injuries; treat the most serious ones first.

Are you alright?
Someone lying motionless on the ground is not necessarily unconscious. Squeeze her hand, call her name, or ask: 'Are you alright? Can you hear me?'

If the casualty responds and speaks, the airway is clear – breathing and circulation are fine. If she is drowsy, turn her into the recovery position (*see* p25) and stay with her. Wait until the emergency service arrives. A casualty in shock or who is bleeding (*see* pp38–9) may be covered with a blanket to conserve body heat.

Monitor responsiveness
Casualties may progress from being conscious to unconscious, their condition either improving or deteriorating fairly rapidly. A fully conscious casualty is able to respond to questions and can hold a conversation. Anything less than that is reason for concern. Main signs of depressed level of consciousness are:
- Drowsy casualty, or one that is difficult to arouse
- Clearly disoriented
- Slurring speech
- Unable to answer your questions correctly

While a casualty is breathing and conscious, try to get information as you wait for medical help.

- Ask what happened. This may give clues to other injuries or conditions that need attention (e.g. if someone has collapsed, it helps to know whether this was the a result of an existing condition such as diabetes). Witnesses may be able to add details.

- Ask if there is pain. Check that site first, and then the rest of the body.
- Use your eyes to search for signs of injury like bruising or swelling. Take note of increased pulse rate or raised temperature.
- Ask whether the casualty has any medical allergies or other conditions requiring special treatment.

MOVING AN INJURED PERSON

As a general rule, resuscitation and first aid should take place where you find the casualty to ensure quick restoration of vital functions (*see* pp22–37) and reduce the risk of complications such as shock, and aggravation of existing injuries. While you commence first aid on the spot, another responsible person should phone for an ambulance or the nearest available doctor.

Severe Injuries

Aggravation of spinal injuries is the main reason why seriously injured casualties should only be moved by trained, equipped medical personnel. Neck and spine injuries are very difficult to detect during first-aid assessment and can easily be converted from minor to disastrous by attempts to move a casualty. Always assume spinal injury in the following situations:

- An unconscious casualty
- Obvious history or signs of head injury
- Injury after a fall from a height, or diving into water
- Sporting injuries (e.g. contact sport or horseriding)
- Casualty complains of a painful neck or back
- Casualty is unable to move arms or legs

Only trained paramedics should move adults with deep, bleeding lacerations or fractures of the lower limb. Children under 20kg (44lbs) with splinted fractures below the knee may be carried for short distances if the injured leg is carefully supported.

If there is obvious risk involved in leaving any injured person where you find them, you must move them, no matter what their injury. For example you must move:
- A burn victim (*see* p52)
- A near-drowning victim (*see* p21)
- Anyone if toxic gas is in the vicinity

Minor injuries and ailments

After first aid has been provided, adults and children with minor injuries may safely be moved to a more comfortable location. Even without injury to a lower limb many casualties are prone to fainting when they stand up, due to a combination of emotional shock, pain and minor blood loss. Remain with the injured persons while they take their first steps.

Injury in remote places

Whether or not to move someone injured at a remote site (apart from the exceptions above) depends on how far you are from help or a telephone. Moving someone is not advised unless you are fit, have no way of summoning help, or can carry the casualty on your back without endangering them.

Two fit adults should be able to carry a casualty for short distances on their interlinked hands. This is useful for conscious people with lower limb injuries and if there is absolutely no risk of spinal injury.

FIRST AID

In order to be helpful and effective, first aid procedures must adhere to certain rules and be performed in specific sequences. The various do's and don'ts are covered in the individual entries dealing with medical emergencies, but ultimately, it all comes down to this: enrol for a recognized first-aid course so that you can rely on your knowledge in any emergency situation. This will enable you to know what to do and to remain calm. If there are no materials to hand, your understanding of what is required will allow you to assess the suitability of items around you in order to improvise. The best advice is: learn the basics. So, attend a recognized course and you could end up saving someone's life one day.

IN THIS SECTION

Assessing a casualty

As with most of the matters involving the human body, it is fairly predictable that no two casualties you will assist as a first responder, will be exactly the same, or require the same type of intervention. Infants are particularly prone to viral infections and to choking, while older children are more prone to asthma and severe injury and elderly people are often troubled by a combination of chronic medical problems, any one of which may cause acute breathing difficulty or circulatory collapse. However, this does not mean that you cannot provide effective first aid without knowing the precise cause of the collapse. Instead, the guidelines for first aid and resuscitation are systematically designed to deal with virtually any instance where you encounter an acutely distressed or unconscious person. The key to being an effective first responder is to follow the basic guidelines in the correct sequences that are recommended in this section of the book: SAFE (*see* below) and ABC (*see* pp22–3).

THE 'SAFE' APPROACH

Whenever you are approaching a casualty who has collapsed for any reason, you should always:
- Summon help immediately – either yourself or by sending another responsible person to call for medical assistance or an emergency service while you attend to the casualty.
- Take precautions to ensure your own safety as well as that of the injured party. This applies especially when attending to casualties injured as a result of road traffic collisions, electricity, fire, toxic inhalation, or any situation where the risk of injury still persists in the vicinity. The SAFE acronym (below) summarizes the correct approach in an easy-to-remember fashion.

 Shout for help: Summon medical assistance or the emergency services immediately.

 Approach with care: Check for surrounding hazards that may also be a danger to yourself.

 Free from danger: Even though we recommend that casualties should not be moved if possible, this precaution must be weighed against any obvious risk, e.g. if a child has been knocked down on a busy street you must move him or her – with all possible care of course – to a safe place before commencing resuscitation.

 Evaluate the ABC: Having taken the above precautions, you are now ready to assess vital functions and commence resuscitation if required.

THE UNCONSCIOUS PERSON

Someone lying motionless on the ground may not be unconscious. Check for response, i.e. establish if a person is conscious by tapping them on the shoulder, or shaking them gently by the shoulder. Call the person's name if you know it, or ask 'Are you alright?' or 'Can you hear me?' If the casualty responds and is able to speak it means that the airway is clear and that breathing and circulation are satisfactory. In this case, stay with him or her and wait for the emergency services to arrive. If the casualty is very drowsy, turn them carefully into the **recovery position** (*see* p25 for adults; p29 for children).

Some common causes of loss of consciousness are **head injury** (*see* pp59–61), **epilepsy** (*see* pp44–5), **stroke** (*see* pp80–1), **meningitis** (*see* pp46–7), and a lack of sufficient oxygen. This is commonly associated with **choking** (*see* pp34–37), **near-drowning** (*see* box on this page) or severe **asthma** (*see* p100).

WHAT TO DO:

- Check the response as described above. If there is none, shout for help.

- Your priority is to **check the ABC** (*see* pp22–3). If the airway is blocked the person will be unable to breathe so your aim is to **open the airway**, then check their breathing and, if necessary, **administer rescue breaths** (*see* p26 for adults; p30 for children; p33 for infants).

- If the casualty is breathing and displays **signs of life** (such as movement and/or coughing) turn them into the recovery position.

- If the person has stopped breathing and shows no signs of life, immediately begin with **chest compressions** (*see* p27 for adults; p31 for children; p33 for infants).

FAINTING

This temporary loss of consciousness results from decreased blood flow to the brain. It commonly

NEAR-DROWNING

Near-drowning victims may be unconscious and will probably be unable to breathe as a result of having been under water. Children can drown in a few centimetres of water because their bodies are top-heavy and this weight, biased towards the upper body makes them overbalance more easily. Infants can drown in a few seconds. For that reason children need constant supervision anywhere near water, even in the bath. If you suspect near-drowning:

- Get the person out of the water immediately.
- Call an ambulance.
- If the casualty is not breathing or unconscious commence **rescue breathing** (*see* p26 for adults and children over 8; p30 for children from 1–8, and p33 for infants from 0–12 months).
- When they are breathing normally, ensure they lie in the recover position.
- It is imperative that you get medical help in all cases of near-drowning.

occurs when someone is feeling very hot, not eating enough, or experiencing an emotional upset, and is caused by sudden slowing of the heart rate. This can be confirmed by checking the pulse rate at the wrist (*see* **circulation** p23). Usually, the only first aid required consists of support, reassurance and a cup of sweetened tea once consciousness returns. Raising the casualty's legs may improve blood flow to the brain and hasten their recovery.

ACCIDENTS HAPPEN

Accident situations in the home are fairly common, small mishaps happen regularly, particularly if your household includes small children. A variety of sound precautions are described in this book that will help to make your home child-friendly (*see* pp130–32).

Procedures for resuscitation

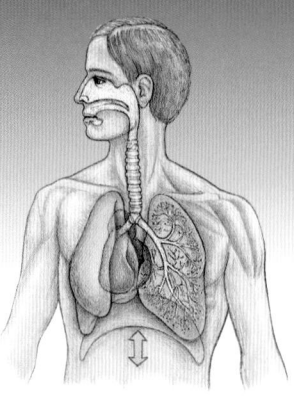

Normal breathing and blood circulation ensure an adequate supply of oxygen and nutrients to all parts of the body. Either or both of these vital functions may fail in an acutely ill or injured casualty. The brain is particularly sensitive and will suffer permanent damage if deprived of oxygen for more than four minutes. Cardiopulmonary resuscitation, a combination of rescue breathing and chest compressions refers to a set of practical skills that enable you to:

The airway, lungs and diaphragm work together to regulate breathing.

- Ensure the casualty has a clear **A**irway to breathe through, and assess the adequacy of **B**reathing and **C**irculation in someone with acute illness or injury (*see* **ABC** below).
- Provide oxygen to casualties who are not able to breathe on their own.
- Establish an artificial heartbeat in someone whose heart is not beating effectively.

The skills described in this section are not enough to turn you into an expert first-aid provider. They should, however, encourage you to enlist for a proper hands-on course offered by a professional organisation.

THE ABC (AIRWAY, BREATHING, CIRCULATION)

CHECK THE AIRWAY

An unconscious person may be unable to breathe if the airway has become obstructed by:

- Kinking, due to abnormal positioning of the head and neck

- The tongue falling back into the throat

- Misplaced dentures

- Food, blood or other foreign matter

Open the airway by lifting the casualty's chin and thus allowing an unobstructed passage to let the air flow in and out of the lungs.

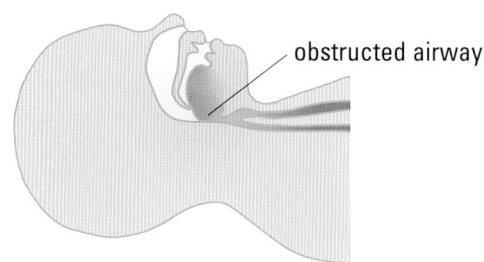

obstructed airway

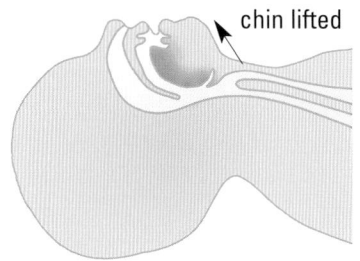

chin lifted

Lift the chin to create an unobstructed passage to the lungs.

RESTORE BREATHING

The normal position of the tongue and the airway can be restored using a combination of the chin-lift and head-tilt (*see* pp24–27 for adults; *see* pp28–31 for children; *see* pp32–3 for infants). Once the airway is cleared:

- Check the mouth for foreign bodies and remove what you can see. Well-fitting dentures that are correctly positioned need not be removed.

- To prevent injuring the person, do not sweep your fingers blindly around inside the mouth or throat.

- When you have opened the airway, the casualty may start breathing unaided. If not, you must give **2 effective rescue breaths** (*see* p26 for adults; p30 for small children; p33 for infants). You can tell that rescue breaths are effective if you see that the casualty's chest rises and falls each time.

CIRCULATION

If the casualty is conscious, meaning that he or she is able to speak and respond to you, or at least able to breathe unaided, then the circulation is in order.

If the person is not responding to you and appears to be uncosncious, you must establish that there are **signs of life**:

- Tap the person on the shoulder, or shake them gently by the shoulder to see if they will respond.

- Call the person's name if you know it, or ask "Can you hear me?", or "Open your eyes."

- Look for visible rising and falling of the chest (indicative that the person is breathing).

- Look for any signs of movement.

To confirm the circulation you can feel for a pulse using the sensitive pads of your index and middle fingers. (Do not use your thumb, because it has its own pulse and may thus mislead you.) Using a watch or clock, record the number of heart beats per minute (the pulse rate), strength of the beats (is the pulse strong or faint?), and the rhythm (is it regular, or irregular?):

- The **radial pulse** is felt on the inside of the wrist roughly at the base of the thumb. Use two or three fingers and press down lightly .

- The **carotid pulse** is felt on the side of the throat between the windpipe and the large neck muscle.

- The **brachial pulse** (used for infants and small children *see* p31) is felt on the inside of the upper arm, just above the elbow.

Normal pulse rate for an adult is between 60 and 80 beats per minute (in fit young people it can be somewhat slower); a young child's pulse is much faster at 140 beats per minute.

If the heart has stopped beating (cardiac arrest) you must try to **restore circulation without delay** using rhythmic chest compression (*see* p27 for adults, p31 for small children; p33 for infants).

UNCONSCIOUS WITH A SUSPECTED NECK INJURY

If there is any possibility of a neck injury in an unconscious casualty, you must restore the airway using the jaw-thrust method. To do this:

- Kneel behind the casualty's head.

- Keeping head, neck and spine aligned, put your hands on either side of the face to support the head. Your fingertips should touch the angles of the jaw; thumbs on cheeks.

- Without tilting the head, lift the jaw forward gently with your fingers to unblock the airway. Listen and look for breathing for 10 seconds.

- If the casualty begins to breathe, maintain support of the head and check breathing and circulation regularly until help arrives. If there is no breathing, begin **rescue breathing** (see p26 adults; p30 children; p33 infants).

RESUSCITATION FOR ADULTS AND OLDER CHILDREN (OVER 8 YEARS)

ASSESSMENT

There are three major scenarios you may encounter. You must first assess which category the casualty falls into (for each of the 'What to do' sections, it is assumed you have classified into the relevant scenario). They may be categorized as follows:

| **1** | unconscious breathing signs of life/circulation | **2** | unconscious not breathing signs of life/circulation | **3** | unconscious not breathing no signs of life/no circulation |

Condition	Adults and children over 8 years of age
Unconscious breathing (*see* below)	Place in **recovery position** (*see* p25) Call an ambulance Ensure airway remains open and normal breathing continues
Unconscious not breathing signs of life/ circulation (*see* p26)	Call an ambulance **Open the airway** (chin lift and head tilt; *see* p26) Listen and look for signs of breathing for 10 seconds Give **2 effective rescue breaths** Check the **circulation** (*see* p23) – refer to Scenario 3 (*see* p27) if necessary Still not breathing: continue rescue breaths at a rate of 10 per minute; check circulation every minute
Unconscious not breathing no signs of life/ no circulation (*see* p27)	No circulation: **15 chest compressions with 2 hands** Continue cycles of **2 breaths to 15 compressions** Continue until breathing resumes or help arrives Place in recovery position if breathing resumes, and monitor carefully

SCENARIO 1 unconscious   breathing   signs of life/circulation

WHAT TO DO:

· Place the casualty in the **recovery position** (*see* opposite).

· Call an ambulance.

· Ensure the airway remains open and that normal breathing continues.

UNCONSCIOUS ADULT (RECOVERY POSITION)

An unconscious casualty who is breathing alone and has normal circulation should be placed in the recovery position. You need to put the person on their side to prevent the tongue from falling back, minimize the risk of vomit being sucked into the lungs and allow you to monitor their breathing and circulation as you wait for help. For treatment **in case of suspected neck or spinal injury** *see* p23.

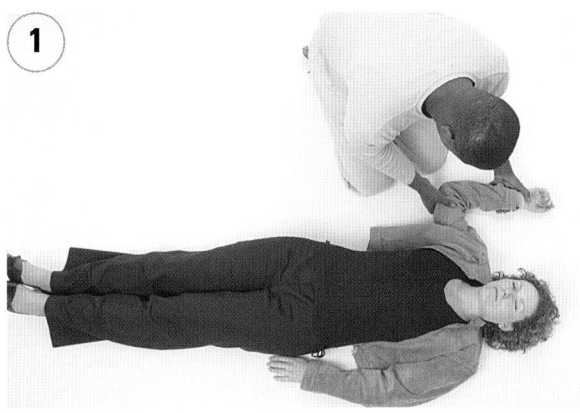

1 Bend the casualty's arm nearest to you at the elbow (±90°), palm up and open.

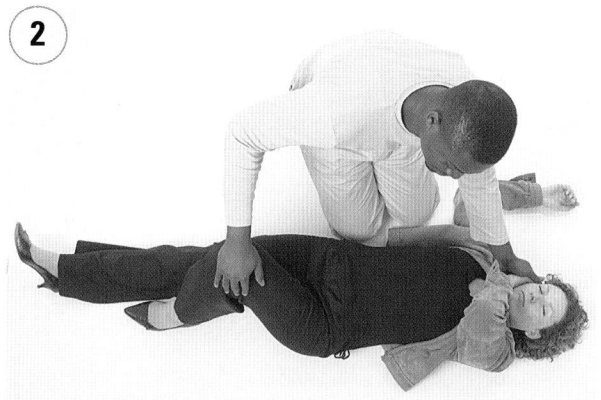

2 Tuck the palm of the hand furthest from you against her cheek. At the same time grasp the knee furthest from you and pull up.

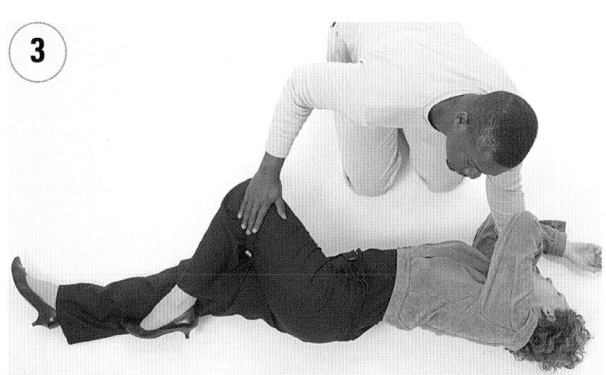

3 Keep her hand on her cheek, pull on her thigh to roll casualty onto the side, facing you.

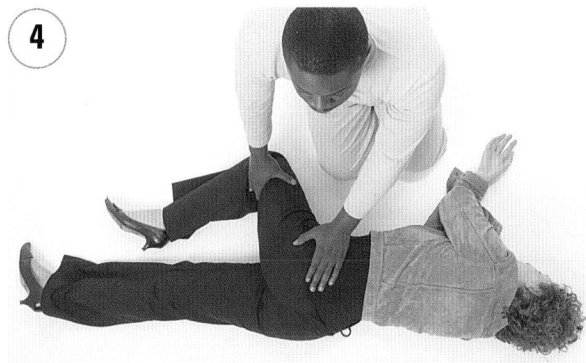

4 Angle her knee at approximately 90°.

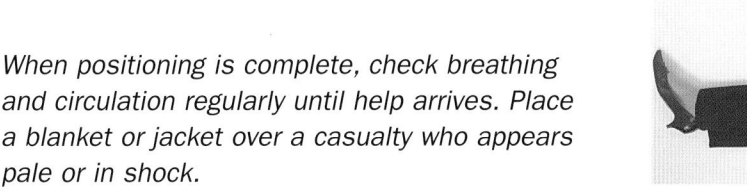

5

When positioning is complete, check breathing and circulation regularly until help arrives. Place a blanket or jacket over a casualty who appears pale or in shock.

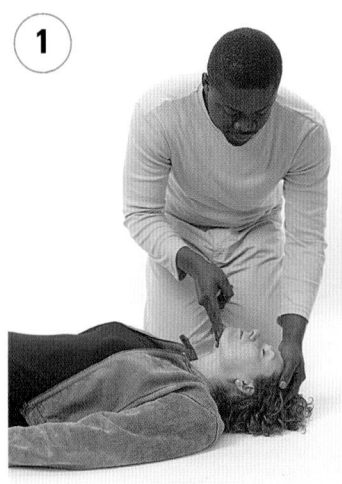

1 Support the casualty's head with the left hand, and tilt the chin up with the fingers of your right hand to open the airway.

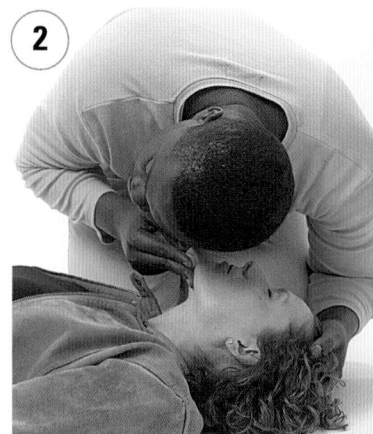

2 For 10 seconds listen for signs of breathing; watch for chest movement.

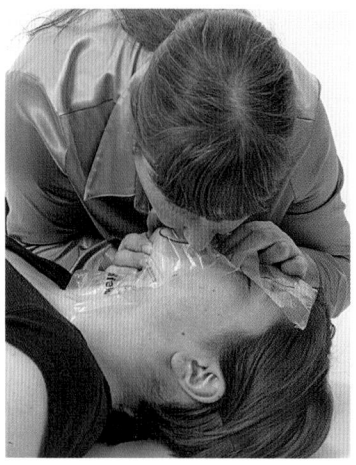

3 Maintain chin lift and pinch the nose shut.

WHAT TO DO:

- Call an ambulance.

- **Open the airway** (*see* step 1).

- Listen and look for **signs of breathing** (*see* step 2). If there is no sign after 10 seconds:

- Open the casualty's mouth, pinch the nose shut and **administer 2 effective rescue breaths** (*see* steps 3 & 4). Then check the **circulation.**

- Continue rescue breaths at a rate of 10 per minute. Check the circulation every minute.

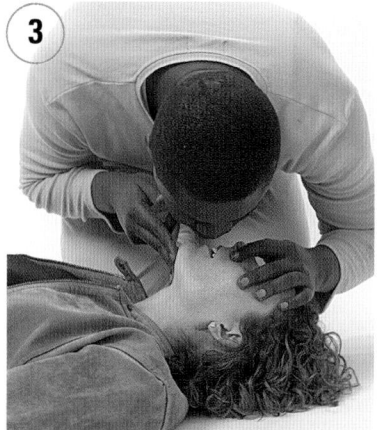

4 Cover casualty's mouth with your own. Keep the airway open. Exhale slowly and firmly. Give 2 effective rescue breaths.

- When the casualty begins to breathe unaided, place in the **recovery position**.

- If you are alone, give 2 effective rescue breaths and then call an ambulance.

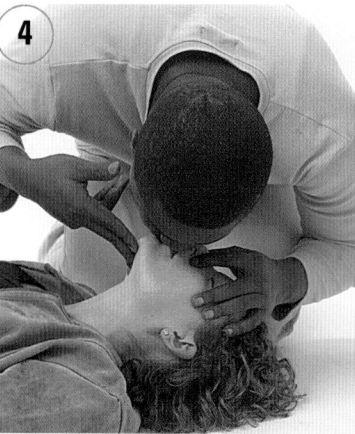

A plastic face shield may be used to prevent infection and for reasons of hygiene. It should be placed over the casualty's face, with the filter over the mouth.

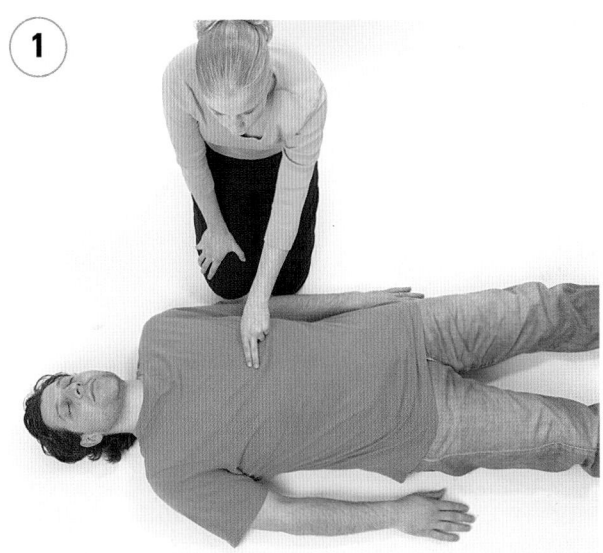

Using two fingers of your left hand locate the notch where the ribs join.

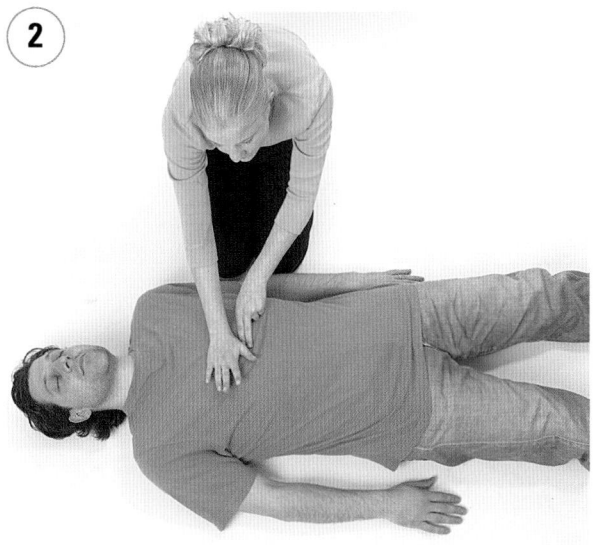

Place your right palm above the notch.

WHAT TO DO:

- Call an ambulance.

- Open the airway; **administer 2 effective rescue breaths** (*see opposite* steps 3 & 4).

- Position your hands as shown (*see* right) and do **15 chest compressions using 2 hands** as follows: keeping your arms straight, lean over the casualty and use your body weight to depress his breastbone to a depth of about 4cm (1½in). Do compressions at a rate of about 100 per minute. Give 2 effective rescue breaths between every 15 compressions.

- Continue cycles of **2 effective rescue breaths for every 15 chest compressions** until breathing resumes or until medical help arrives.

- Place in **recovery position** if casualty begins to breathe unaided.

- If you are alone, do cycles of 2 rescue breaths to 15 chest compressions for one minute, then call an ambulance.

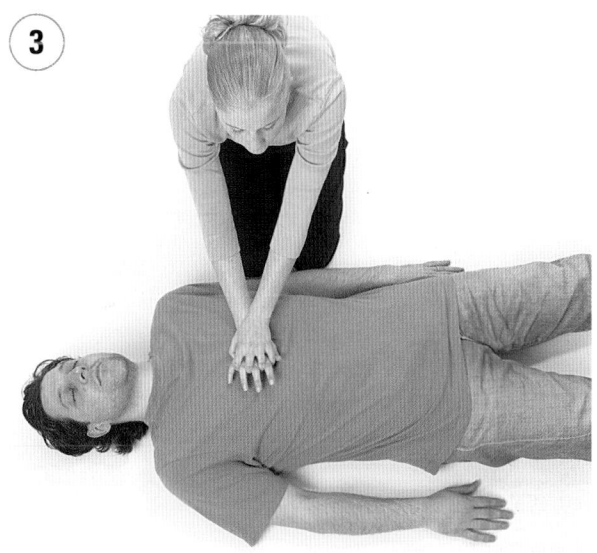

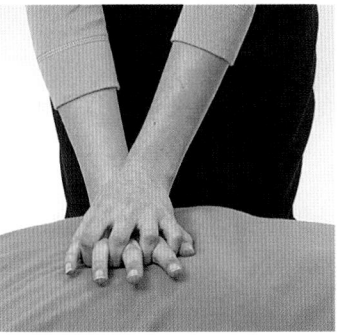

Place the heel of your left hand over the right so that your fingers can interlock (see above and right). Do the chest compressions keeping your arms straight.

Chest compressions for adults and older children

RESUSCITATION FOR CHILDREN (1–8 YEARS)

ASSESSMENT

There are three major scenarios you may encounter. You must first assess which category the casualty falls into (for each of the 'What to do' sections, it is assumed you have classified into the relevant scenario). They may be categorized as follows:

1 unconscious
breathing
signs of life/circulation

2 unconscious
not breathing
signs of life/circulation

3 unconscious
not breathing
no signs of life/no circulation

Condition	Children 1–8 years of age
Unconscious breathing (*see* below)	Place in **recovery position** (*see* opposite) Call an ambulance Ensure airway remains open and that normal breathing continues
Unconscious not breathing signs of life/ circulation (*see* p30)	Call an ambulance **Open the airway** (chin lift and head tilt – *see* p30) Listen and look for signs of breathing for 10 seconds Give **2 effective rescue breaths** Check the **circulation** (*see* p23 and p31) – refer to Scenario 3 (*see* p31) if necessary
Unconscious not breathing no signs of life/ no circulation (*see* p31)	No circulation: **5 chest compressions with 1 hand** Continue cycles of **1 breath to 5 chest compressions** Continue until normal breathing resumes of help arrives Place in recovery position if breathing resumes, and monitor carefully

SCENARIO 1   unconscious   breathing   signs of life/circulation

WHAT TO DO:

· Place the casualty in the **recovery position** (*see* opposite).

· Call an ambulance.

· Ensure the airway remains open and that normal breathing continues.

UNCONSCIOUS CHILD (RECOVERY POSITION)

An unconscious casualty who is breathing alone and has normal circulation should be placed in the recovery position. You need to put the child on its side to prevent the tongue from falling back, minimize the risk of vomit being sucked into the lungs and allow you to monitor their breathing and circulation as you wait for help. For treatment **in case of suspected neck or spinal injury** *see* p23.

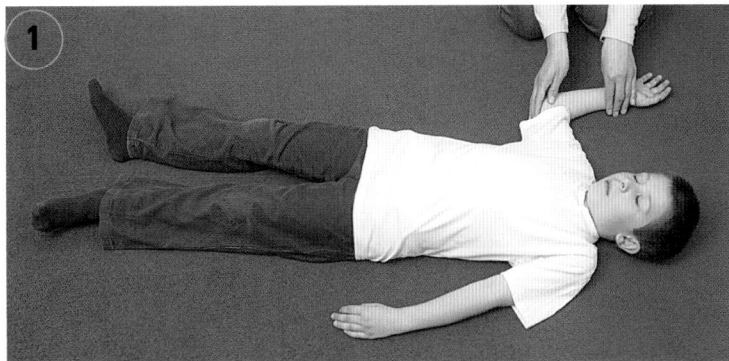

Angle the right arm next to the child's head at approximately 90°.

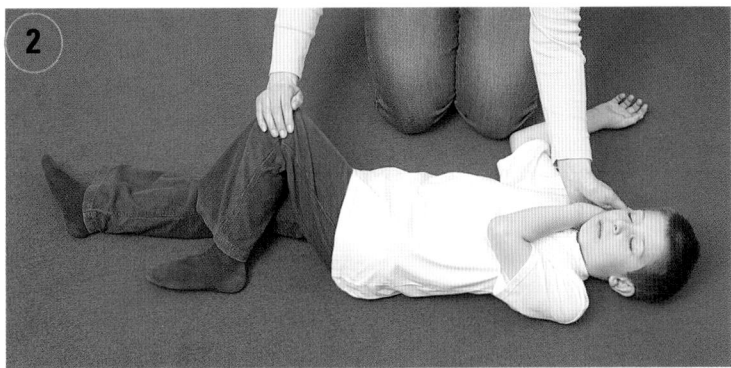

Position the right hand as shown and bring the left across the chest towards you to, palm showing out and the back of the hand resting against the right cheek. Bend the left leg at the knee as shown.

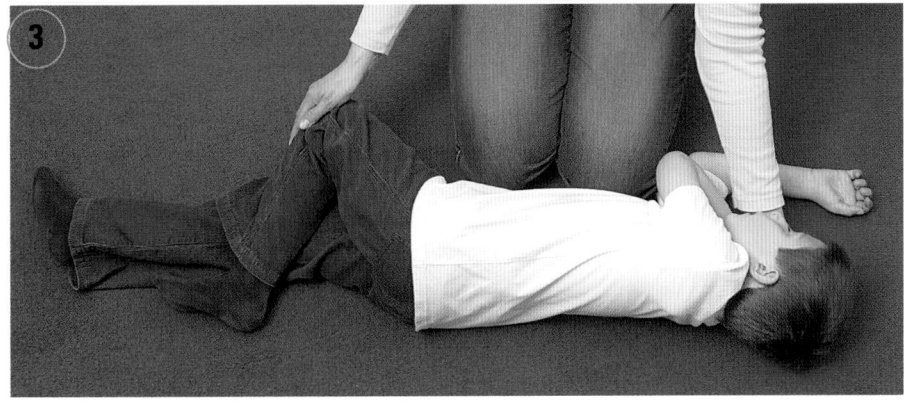

You can now move the child into the recovery position with your one hand stabilizing the head to protect the neck, while you use the other to bend the knee. Then gently roll the trunk over. Ensure that airway remains open and the casualty continues to breathe normally.

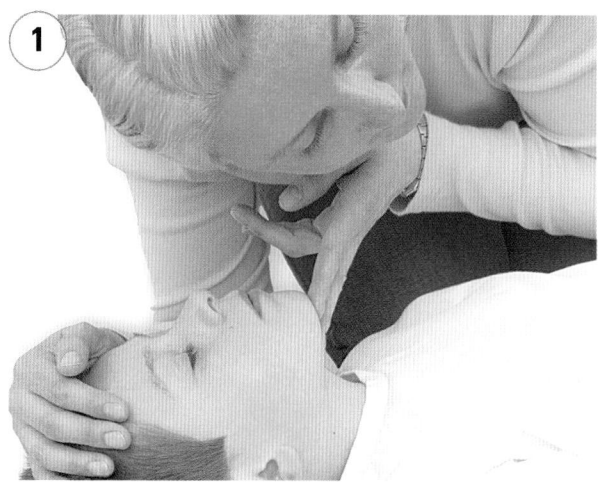

Gently lift the chin using two fingers of one hand while the other holds the head steady. Listen and feel for signs of breathing for 10 seconds.

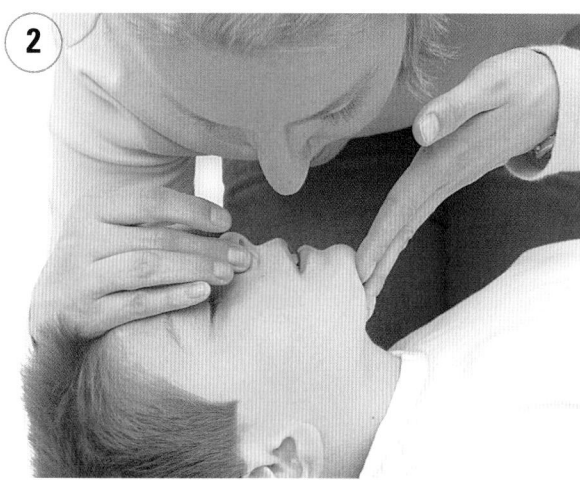

Maintaining the chin lift and position of the head, gently pinch the nose shut with the fingers of your other hand and inhale.

Open the casualty's mouth, cover his mouth with yours and give 2 effective rescue breaths.

WHAT TO DO:

- Call an ambulance.

- **Open the airway** using the chin lift and head tilt (*see* step 1).

- Listen and look for **signs of breathing** for about 10 seconds.

- If there is no sign of breathing, open casualty's mouth, pinch his nose shut and **administer 2 effective rescue breaths** (*see* step 3).

- Check the **circulation**.

- Continue rescue breaths at a rate of 1 every 3 seconds (20 per minute) until the child begins to breathe unaided or until help arrrives. Check the **circulation** every minute.

- Place the casualty in the **recovery position** if they begin to breathe normally.

- If you are alone, give 2 effective rescue breaths then call an ambulance.

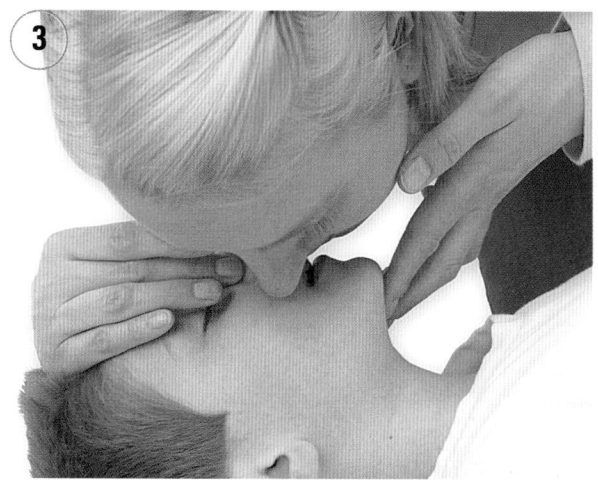

WHAT TO DO:

- Call an ambulance.

- Open the airway (*see* left, step 1) and make 5 attempts to give **2 effective rescue breaths** (*see opposite*, step 3).

- Position your hand over the lower half of the breastbone as shown (below) and do **5 compressions using the heel of one hand**. Keeping your arm straight, lean over the child and press down on the child's chest. Keep your fingers lifted up. Do compressions at a rate of about 100 per minute.

- Give **1 effective rescue breath between every 5 compressions** and continue this until breathing resumes or medical help arrives.

- Place in **recovery position** if casualty begins to breathe unaided.

- If you are alone: cycles of 1 breath to 5 compressions for one minute, then call an ambulance.

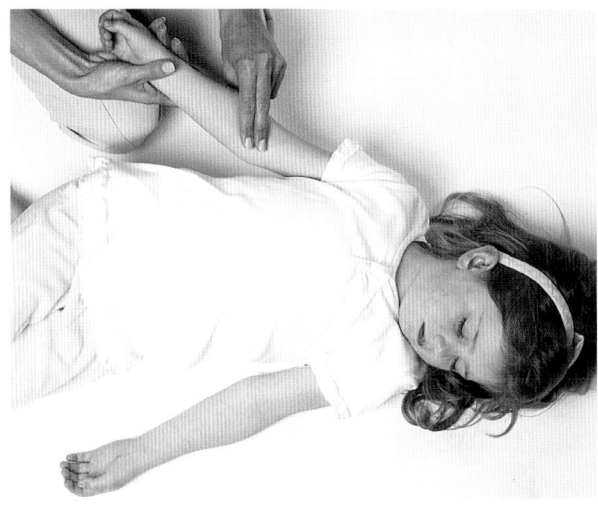

In small children and infants the pulse can be felt at the brachial artery. Use the sensitive pads of your fingers to feel it. A child's pulse is usually around 140 beats per minute, a rate much higher than that of adults.

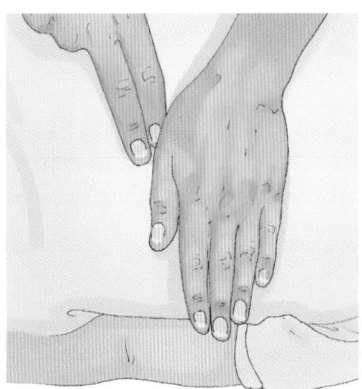

Locate the breastbone using two fingers; position your other hand so that the heel of your palm lies directly over the lower half of the breastbone.

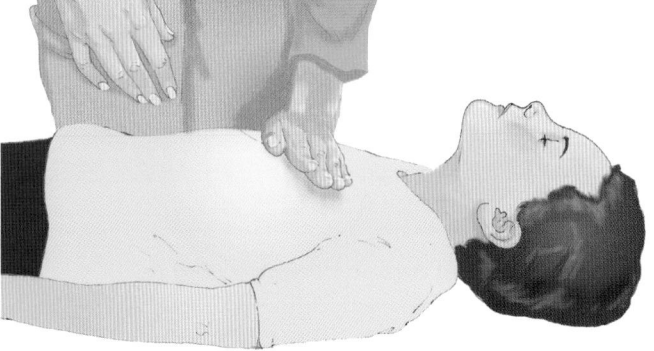

Using only the heel of your one hand, compress the child's chest to a depth of about 3cm (1in) in a quick movement. For every 5 chest compressions, give 1 effective rescue breath. Do about 100 compressions per minute, alternating with rescue breaths as described, until the child begins to breathe spontaneously and manages to carry on breathing unaided, or until medical help arrives.

RESUSCITATION FOR INFANTS (0–12 MONTHS)

ASSESSMENT

There are three major scenarios you may encounter. You must first assess which category the casualty falls into (for each of the 'What to do' sections, it is assumed you have classified into the relevant scenario). They may be categorized as follows:

1 unconscious
breathing
signs of life/circulation

2 unconscious
not breathing
signs of life/circulation

3 unconscious
not breathing
no signs of life/no circulation

Condition	Infants 0–12 months of age
Unconscious breathing (*see* below)	Hold in **recovery position** (*see* below) Call an ambulance Ensure airway remains open and normal breathing continues
Unconscious not breathing signs of life/ circulation (*see* opposite)	Call an ambulance **Open the airway** (chin lift and head tilt – *see* opposite) Listen and look for signs of breathing for 10 seconds Give **2 effective rescue breaths** Check the **circulation** (*see* p23 and p31) – refer to Scenario 3 (*see* opposite) if necessary
Unconscious not breathing no signs of life/ no circulation (*see* opposite)	If no circulation give **5 chest compressions using only 2 fingers** Continue cycles of **1 breath to 5 chest compressions** Continue until normal breathing resumes or help arrives If normal breathing resumes place in recovery position (*see* below) and monitor carefully

SCENARIO **1** unconscious · breathing · signs of life/circulation

WHAT TO DO:

· Hold the infant in the **recovery position** (*see* right).

· Call an ambulance.

· Ensure the airway remains open and that normal breathing continues.

Cradle the infant in your arms. Your one hand should support his head and hold it slightly lower thant the rest of the body, while the other hand supports the infant's back.

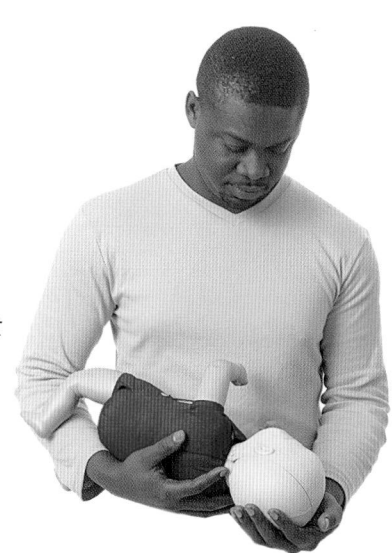

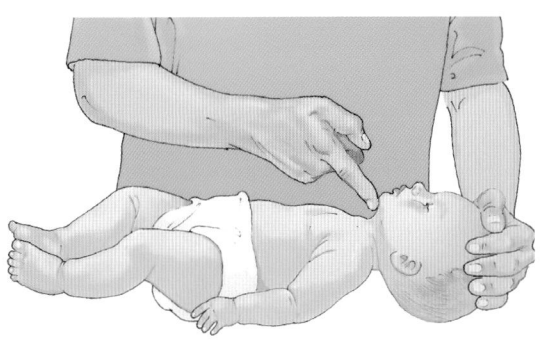 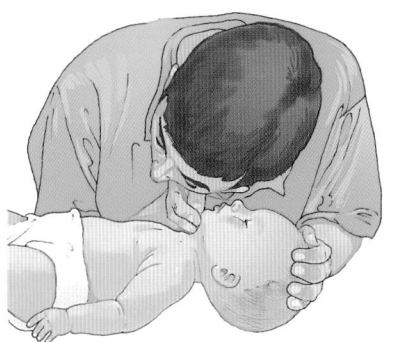

With your left hand, stabilize the infant's head as shown. Then gently tilt the chin up with your right index finger. For 10 seconds listen for sounds of breathing.

WHAT TO DO:

- Call an ambulance.

- Open the airway; give **2 effective rescue breaths** (*see* right); check the **circulation**.

- Do rescue breaths at a rate of 1 breath every 3 seconds (20 per minute) until infant starts to breathe or help arrives. Check the circulation every minute.

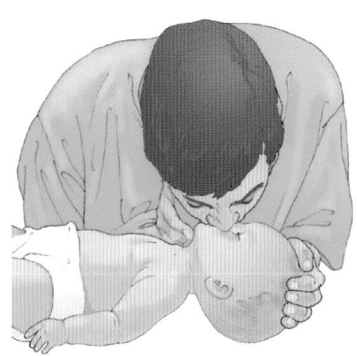

- If you are alone, give 2 effective rescue breaths then call an ambulance.

- When the infant begins to breathe unaided, hold in recovery position (*see* opposite).

SCENARIO 3 unconscious   not breathing   no signs of life/no circulation

WHAT TO DO:

- Call an ambulance.

- Open airway and **give 2 effective rescue breaths**.

- **Using 2 fingers do 5 compressions** (at a rate of 100 per minute) to a depth of 2cm (¾in).

- Give **1 effective rescue breath for every 5 compressions** until breathing resumes or help arrives.

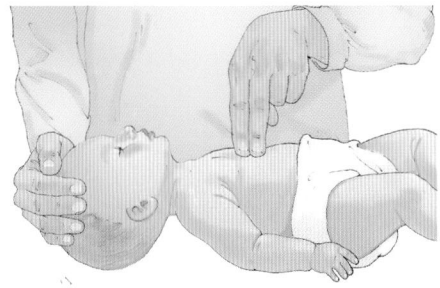

- If you are alone do cycles of 1 breath per 5 chest compressions for one minute, then call ambulance, taking the infant with you.

Put the tips of index and middle finger on breast-bone, one finger below an imaginary line joining the nipples.

Choking

Choking is caused by an obstruction of the upper airway, commonly as a result of food becoming impacted. In some cases, a coughing spell is enough to expel a foreign body from the airway. However, even small objects may lodge firmly in the narrow airway of an infant or small child, in which case you may have to use the techniques described here to clear the airway. The upper airway can also become obstructed by tissue swelling caused by **allergy** (*see* p101), or severe infection. In such cases, treatment of underlying causes is required. Techniques described here are designed to help the casualty expel a foreign body by creating a high-pressure wave inside the lungs, rather like an artificial cough. If you suspect choking in an unconscious casualty, first attend to the ABC (*see* pp22–3). Use the techniques described here only if you are unable to give effective rescue breaths.

Condition	Adults and children over 8 years of age
Suspected choking	Up to 5 back blows – check the mouth and remove any obstruction Up to 5 abdominal thrusts – check the mouth and remove any obstruction Do 3 cycles of back blows and abdominal thrusts If breathing: **open airway** and remove visible foreign matter (*see* p22) place in **recovery position** (*see* p25) If not breathing, commence **resuscitation sequence** (*see* pp22–27)

SYMPTOMS

In someone who is unconscious or struggling to breathe, you should consider choking as the cause whenever:
- a healthy adult or child has a sudden coughing spell, and then struggles to breathe.
- you find other foreign bodies, i.e. peanuts or small toy parts, near the casualty.
- a casualty who is coughing or struggling to breathe may point at his neck to indicate that something is stuck in the throat.
- resuscitation remains ineffective despite the head tilt and chin lift being correctly applied.

Common causes of airway obstruction

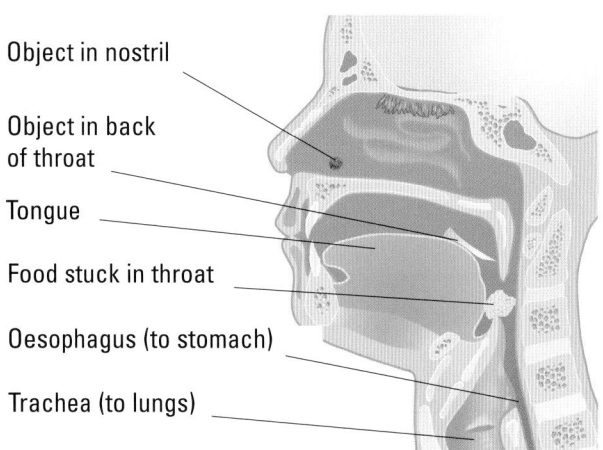

Object in nostril

Object in back of throat

Tongue

Food stuck in throat

Oesophagus (to stomach)

Trachea (to lungs)

FIRST AID FOR CHOKING ADULTS AND OLDER CHILDREN (OVER 8 YEARS)

Use a combination of back blows and abdominal thrusts for an adult or older child who seems to be choking and is unable to breathe or cough up the foreign body themselves. Do 3 cycles of the entire procedure then **call an ambulance if there is no improvement**. Follow this with 5 attempts to give 2 effective rescue breaths. If still unsuccessful, begin resuscitation (*see* pp22–27).

BACK BLOWS
WHAT TO DO:

· Using the heel of your hand, give up to 5 firm back blows between the shoulder blades.

· Carefully check in the casualty's mouth for obvious obstructions. Do not probe blindly.

· Remove the obstruction.

· If this does not help, do abdominal thrusts too.

ABDOMINAL THRUST
WHAT TO DO:

If back blows fail to dislodge the obstruction, do up to 5 abdominal thrusts. These can be done with the person standing, seated on your lap, or – in a choking casualty who has lost consciousness – lying flat on the ground. If at any stage during this sequence the casualty begins to breathe, check the mouth and clear away any visible foreign object.

· Place one fisted hand midway between the navel and the breastbone and place the palm of your free hand over the fist.

· Using both hands, thrust firmly inwards and upwards towards the chest up to five times.

· If there is no relief after 3 cycles of back blows and abdominal thrusts, call an ambulance.

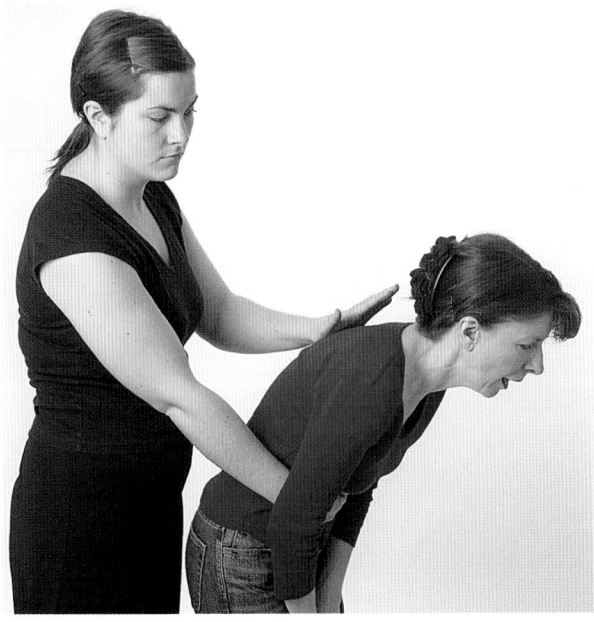

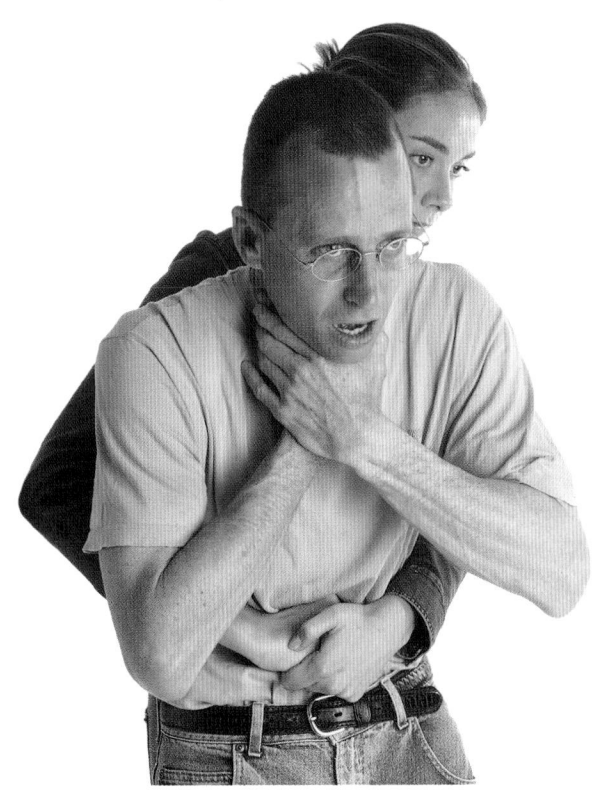

FIRST AID FOR CHOKING CHILDREN (1–8 YEARS)

Condition	Children 1–8 years of age
Suspected choking	Up to 5 back blows – check the mouth and remove any obstruction Up to 5 chest thrusts – check the mouth and remove any obstruction Up to 5 abdominal thrusts – check the mouth and remove any obstruction Do 3 cycles of back blows, chest thrusts and abdominal thrusts If breathing: **open airway** and remove visible foreign matter (*see* p28) place in **recovery position** (*see* p29) If not breathing, commence **resuscitation sequence** (*see* p30)

Use a combination of back blows, chest thrusts and abdominal thrusts for small children who show signs of choking and are unable to breathe or cough up the foreign body themselves. Do 3 cycles of the entire procedure then **call an ambulance if there is no improvement**. Follow this with 5 attempts to give 2 effective rescue breaths. If still unsuccessful, begin resuscitation (see pp28–31). You can stand, sit or kneel behind the child to perform these procedures.

BACK BLOWS
WHAT TO DO:

- Seated or kneeling, do back blows with the child lying face down across your thighs.

- Give up to five back blows between the shoulder blades with the palm of your hand.

- Check the mouth for any obvious obstructions, such as a particle of food and remove without probing blindly.

- If there is no relief, do 5 chest thrusts.

CHEST THRUSTS

If the back blows fail to dislodge the obstruction, do up to 5 chest thrusts.

- Cover one fist with your other hand, place against the lower part of the breastbone and press inwards up to five times.

- Check the mouth for obstructions, and remove.

ABDOMINAL THRUSTS

If the chest thrusts fail to dislodge the obstruction, do up to 5 abdominal thrusts.

- Place one fist against the abdomen, cover with your free palm and thrust firmly inwards and upwards up to five times.

- If the casualty begins to breathe, check the mouth and clear away any visible foreign object.

- If there is no relief after 3 cycles of back blows, chest and abdominal thrusts call an ambulance.

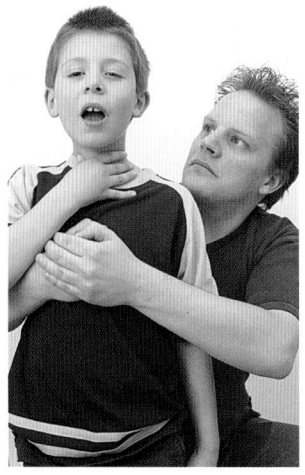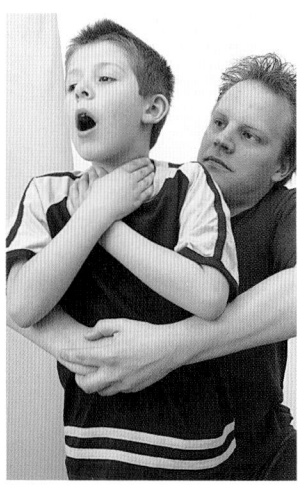

Chest thrust *Abdominal thrust*

FIRST AID FOR CHOKING INFANTS (0–12 MONTHS)

Condition	Infants 0–12 months of age
Suspected choking	Up to 5 back blows – check the mouth and remove any obstruction Up to 5 chest thrusts – check the mouth and remove any obstruction Do 3 cycles of back blows and chest thrusts If breathing: **open airway** and remove visible foreign matter (*see* p33) hold in **recovery position** (*see* p32) If not breathing, commence **resuscitation sequence** (*see* p33)

Use a combination of back blows and chest thrusts for infants who show signs of choking. Do 3 cycles of the entire procedure then **call an ambulance if there is no improvement**. Follow this with 5 attempts to give 2 effective rescue breaths. If unsuccessful, begin resuscitation (*see* pp32–3). And note please: NEVER DO ABDOMINAL THRUSTS ON AN INFANT.

BACK BLOWS
WHAT TO DO:

- Hold infant face down and tilted head-down along your arm, resting your arm on your thigh for support.

- Using heel of your free hand, deliver up to 5 blows between infant's shoulder blades.

- Turn infant over onto your other arm. Check its mouth and remove any foreign object.

- If this does not help, do chest thrusts.

CHEST THRUSTS
WHAT TO DO:

- Turn the infant face-up, with its head lower than its hips.

- With the tips of two fingers, give 5 chest thrusts over the breastbone (depress about 2cm; ¾in). Thrusts should be about three seconds apart.

- Check the mouth and clear away foreign object. If the infant does not breathe after 3 cycles, call an ambulance immediately.

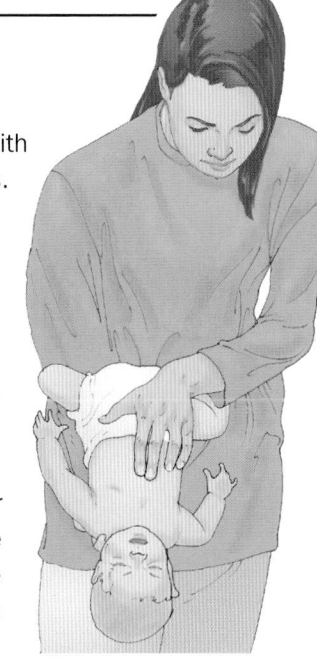

⚠ CAUTION

- **NEVER do abdominal thrusts on infants.**

If the infant fails to breath normally after 5 back blows and 5 chest thrusts:
- **Open the airway** (*see* p33); remove visible foreign matter from the mouth.
- If they stop breathing altogether, maintain the airway correctly and give up to 5 **rescue breaths** (*see* p33).
- If rescue breaths are ineffective, repeat the back blows and chest thrusts in cycles of five and call an ambulance.

Bleeding

Bleeding (loss of blood) occurs either externally – through a break in the skin, or through a natural opening such as the mouth. Substantial or ongoing blood loss will inevitably lead to **shock** (*see* p40), with particular risk of damage to the brain and kidneys. The aim of the first-aid provider is to recognize severe bleeding and control it so that: the flow of blood is effectively stemmed, there is a minimal risk of infection and the casualty does not go into shock from loss of blood – *see also* the **DO NOT** box on page 45. It is essential to get the injured person to a doctor or hospital as soon as possible.

TREATMENT

·   **Call an ambulance** if the bleeding appears to be very severe.

·   For deep wounds that are free of foreign objects, **stop the bleeding** by applying firm pressure on the wound using a sterile pad or clean cloth. If blood soaks through do not remove the pad, but simply place a second one over it. If you have nothing available with which to make a pad, use your hand. Be sure to maintain the pressure until help arrives.

·   Examine the wound carefully to see whether there is any foreign object, such as a shard of glass, embedded in it. If there is DO NOT REMOVE it.

TIP

Use surgical gloves to prevent infection. (HIV and viral hepatitis can be transmitted if infected blood makes contact with broken skin.) If you have no gloves, wash your hands well before and after first aid, using an antiseptic soap or solution.

Instead, place a sterile piece of gauze or cloth gently over the embedded object and bandage around it (*see* p86).

·   Elevate the limb, either by holding it up, or using any handy object (such as a chair, or a rock) to support it. This elevation will reduce the bleeding by diverting blood from the wound, and will also prevent the casualty from going into shock by directing more blood towards the brain.

·   Reassure the casualty and get him or her to sit comfortably or **lie down** if they appear slightly disoriented and look pale and distressed. Monitor the casualty closely for signs of **shock** (*see* pp40–41) while you attend to the wound.

·   When you have controlled the bleeding, leave the first pad in position and **bandage** the wound (*see* p39). If the wound bleeds heavily through the first and second pad while you bandage, discard both pads and begin again with a fresh pad pressed firmly to the wound to staunch the flow of blood. It is imperative that you control the bleeding.

·   If necessary, get the casualty to lie down. This reduces the chance of fainting by increasing the blood flow to the brain. Raise the legs to maintain blood pressure (*see* p41).

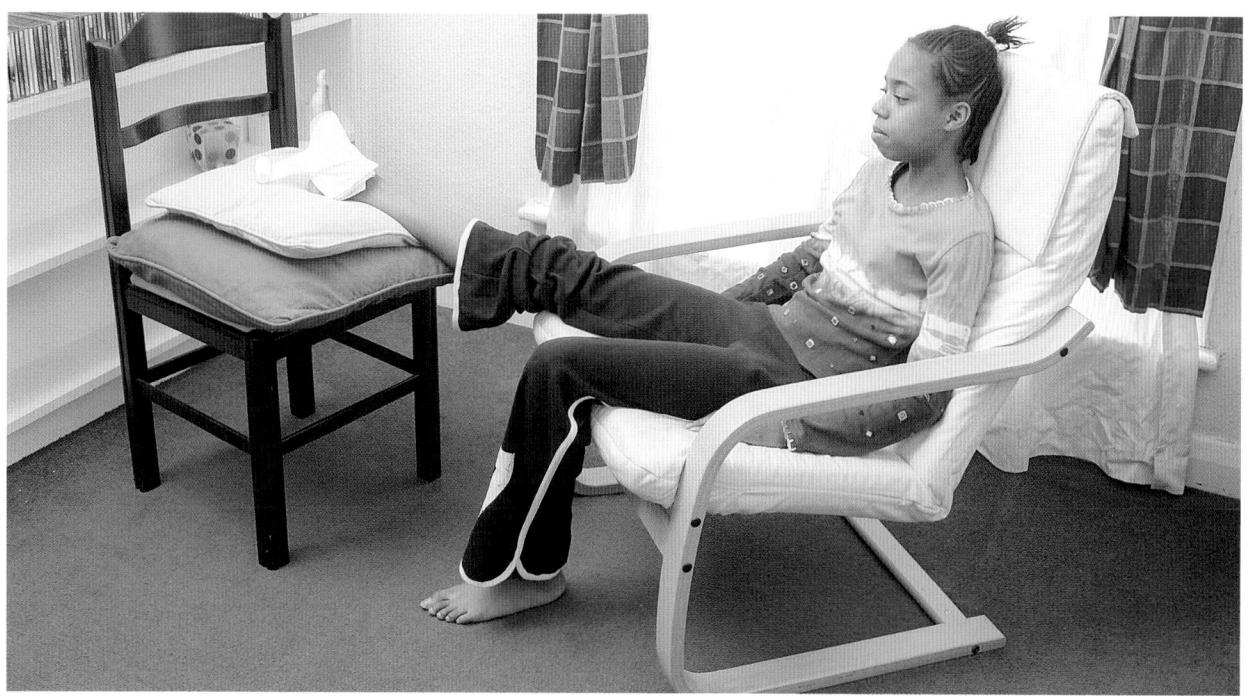

When you have stopped the bleeding and bandaged the wound, get the casualty to lie down or sit comfortably and elevate the limb.

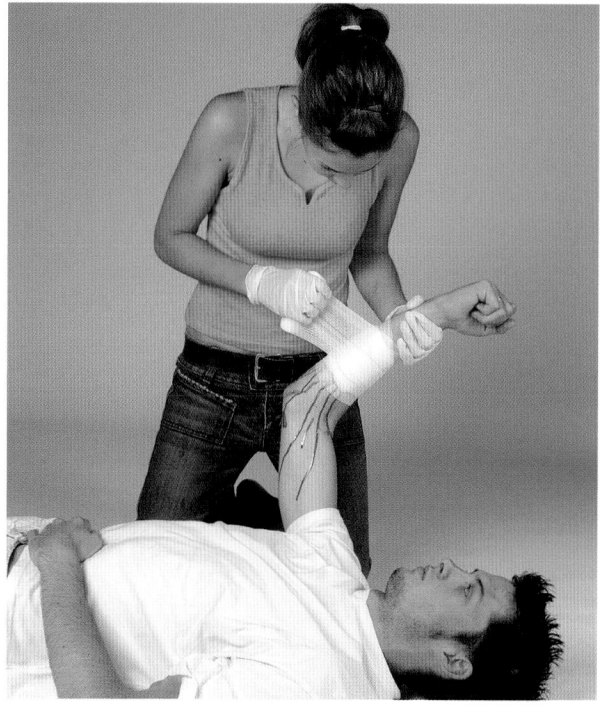

Raise the limb to decrease blood flow to the wound and increase blood flow to the brain. Apply apply direct pressure to the area.

X DO NOT

- **remove an embedded object**, such as a piece of glass, or a knife, for example. If it has punctured an organ, removing it could do more damage and increase the amount of bleeding. Make a **ring bandage** (*see* p86) around the object by using two or more tightly rolled-up bandages as supports around the embedded object to prevent it from being pressed any deeper into the wound. Once the support stays are in place, you can bandage on and around them without touching the embedded object or the wound itself, while at the same time maintaining pressure on the wound to staunch the flow of blood.

Shock

Shock results when the regular, healthy blood flow to tissues and organs is reduced to a dangerously low level. It can be caused by a variety of conditions, including sudden **bleeding** (*see* p38), **heart attack** (*see* below and pp78–9), **anaphylactic shock** (*see* p42), **burns** (*see* p52), and damage to the nervous system (**spinal cord injuries**, *see* p74) and even **head injury** (*see* pp59–61). If shock is not treated rapidly enough, vital organs, such as the heart, kidneys and brain, may suffer damage and fail. The body reacts to shock by directing blood away from the extremities and towards the vital organs. Always treat shock as an urgent medical emergency as the effects can worsen very quickly and may require **rescue breaths** (*see* p26) and/or **resuscitation** (*see* pp22–37).

SYMPTOMS

These vary, depending on what caused the shock, but may include the following:
- Paleness (pallor)
- Moist, cool, clammy skin
- Nausea and vomiting
- A rapid and/or irregular pulse that turns gradually weaker
- Shallow breathing
- Repeated yawning and/or sighing
- Blue-tinged lips and fingernails
- Agitation, anxiety or confusion
- Restlessness
- Thirst
- Fainting
- Unconsciousness
- Chest pain
- Profuse sweating

CAUSES
- Bleeding or severe dehydration following a serious injury (hypovolemic shock).
- Heart attack or heart failure (cardiogenic shock).
- Allergic reactions (anaphylactic shock).
- Spinal cord injuries (neurogenic shock).
- Loss of body fluids as a result of burns, severe diarrhoea or vomiting.

TREATMENT
- If you suspect someone may be suffering from shock, summon medical assistance immediately.

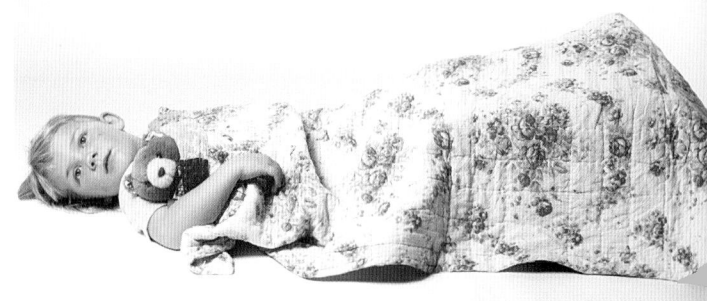

Lying the patient down with their feet raised allows the blood to circulate more easily.

Treat all obvious injuries (burns, fractures and/or bleeding) and be sure to **monitor the vital signs** (*see* pp22–3) and treat as appropriate until medical assistance arrives.

· **If the casualty is conscious** and you are sure there is no injury to the head, neck, spine or legs, lay them flat on their back on the floor with their feet raised about 30cm (12in), or above the level of the heart.

· **If a head or spinal injury is suspected**, do not attempt to move the casualty at all – they should remain in the same position as found until medical assistance arrives.

· **If a casualty vomits or drools**, turn their head to one side to prevent choking through the inhalation of vomit into the lungs. If there is an injury to the head or spine, hold the casualty's head still in relation to their body and roll them onto their side. Place supporting material under the head to keep it in the same position relative to the body.

· **Loosen tight clothing** and cover the casualty with a blanket or garment for warmth.

· **Reassure the casualty**, and give appropriate first aid for any wounds, injuries, or illnesses.

· **Do not give a shocked casualty anything to eat or drink**. Moisten the lips if they are thirsty.

PREVENTION

As with other emergencies, early recognition of the underlying cause and ensuring immediate medical care will limit the severity of shock.

Controlling external bleeding effectively in an injured person will assist the body's own mechanisms to maintain a normal blood pressure and thereby prevent shock from deteriorating to a level where the person's life is at risk.

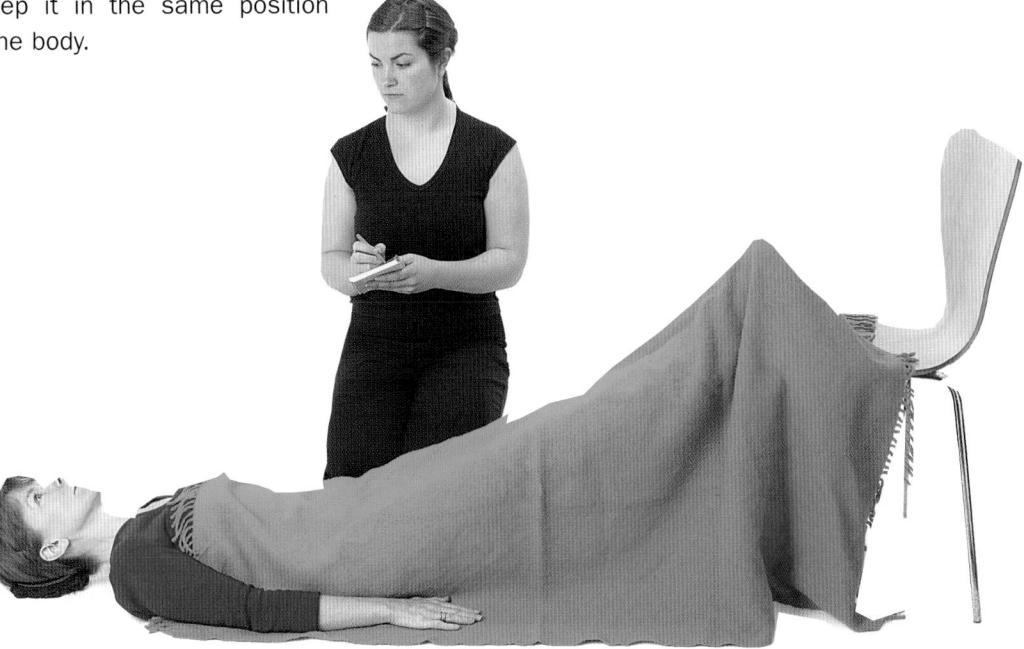

While you are waiting for medical help to arrive make the casualty is covered with a warm blanket and lying as comfortable as possible. Monitor the vital signs regularly and record your findings for rate of breathing, responsiveness and pulse.

Anaphylactic Shock

Anaphylaxis (anaphylactic shock) is a rare but severe hypersensitivity (allergic) reaction that occurs when a person's immune system recognizes a particular substance as a threat to the whole body. The reaction spreads rapidly throughout the body, causing blood pressure to drop suddenly and narrowing the airways, making breathing difficult. Anaphylaxis can be fatal unless immediate treatment is available.

SYMPTOMS

The symptoms usually develop very quickly and may include the following:

- Difficulty in breathing
- Wheezing, or abnormal, high-pitched breathing sounds
- Tightness in the chest and throat
- Itchy red skin rash
- Swollen face, lips and tongue
- Anxiety or confusion
- Light-headedness, fainting, loss of consciousness
- Abdominal pain, cramping, diarrhoea
- Nausea and vomiting
- Nasal congestion or coughing
- Palpitations (sensation of feeling the heart beat)
- Rapid or weak pulse
- Slurred speech
- Blueness of the skin, including the lips or nail beds

CAUSES

Extreme allergic reaction to a specific substance. Common allergens include insect stings; allergies to certain foods, such as shellfish, nuts or strawberries; or to specific medicines, such as penicillin (*see also* **allergies** p101).

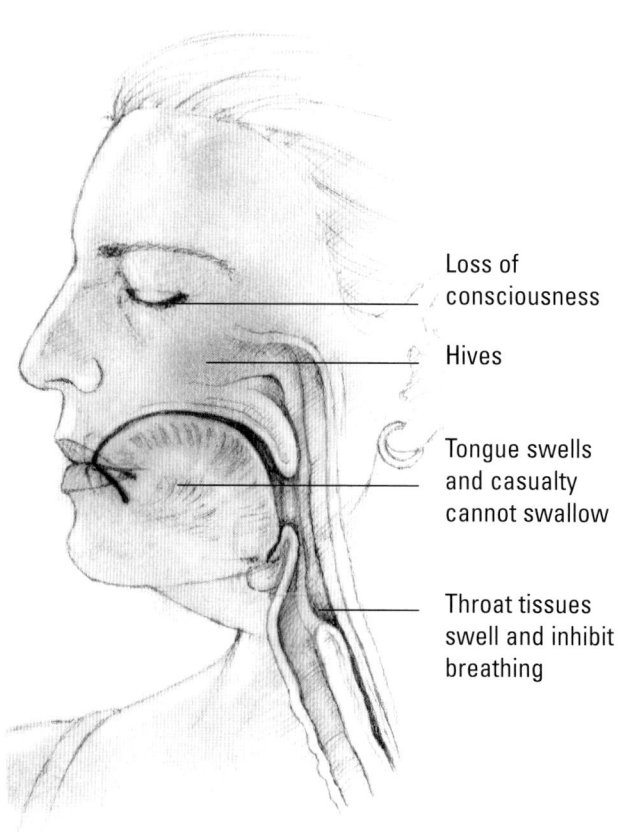

Loss of consciousness

Hives

Tongue swells and casualty cannot swallow

Throat tissues swell and inhibit breathing

TREATMENT

- **Get to a doctor or call an ambulance right away**. Anaphylaxis can be fatal unless promptly treated.
- While waiting, if the casualty is conscious, help him into a sitting position to ease breathing. If the casualty has an **Epipen** (adrenaline or epinephrine syringe), help him to administer it to the thigh muscle, through clothing if necessary.
- If the casualty loses consciousness, carry out **rescue breaths** (*see* p26) if necessary.
- **Do not leave the casualty alone**, except when you go to call an ambulance.

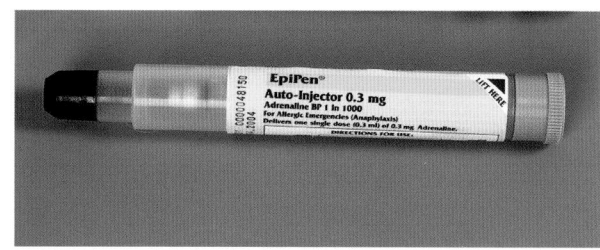

If you suffer from a severe allergy, you should always carry an adrenaline-filled syringe. In the event of an anaphylactic reaction, the adrenaline should be injected into your thigh muscle.

CAUTION

- If you are alone when you have symptoms that suggest you may be having an anaphylactic reaction, contact your doctor or an emergency service immediately and explain what is happening to you. Don't drive yourself to the emergency room – the symptoms may become more pronounced en route and cause you to have an accident.

PREVENTION

People who have a known sensitivity to particular allergens should always wear a medical alert tag so the correct treatment can be given in an emergency. They should also ask their doctor to prescribe an emergency kit to keep at home. (Such kits normally contain antihistamines and a syringe of adrenaline.)

The best prevention is to avoid exposure to known allergens. For example, if you are allergic to bee stings, wear long pants and long-sleeved tops when you are working in the garden or taking part in any outdoor activities.

Food allergy sufferers should read packaging labels, and enquire about the ingredients used when ordering in a restaurant, stating clearly that they are allergic to a particular food.

A clearly visible Medic Alert tag must be worn at all times. It will provide medical personnel with details of your allergies in the event that you are unable to speak for yourself. This is especially important if you are allergic to penicillin or other medications which may be given in an emergency situation .

Convulsions and seizures

A seizure can be alarming to witness: it may last anything from 30 seconds to a couple of minutes, and involve the whole body or just one part. In severe cases, there may be violent muscle contractions and relaxations triggered by spontaneous electrical activity in the casualty's brain, causing them to convulse. Nothing can be done to end a seizure. All you can do is wait it out and try to ensure that the person does not suffer an injury by slamming a limb into a table, for example. If a seizure lasts longer than two minutes or so, or one seizure follows another in quick succession without the casualty regaining consciousness between each one, you have a medical emergency on your hands, as the person will be unable to breathe normally for the duration of the seizure. Summon assistance immediately and note the duration and severity of the seizure, what movements the casualty made, and with which limbs, if there was a loss of bladder control, any eye or head movements, and whether the casualty displayed different levels of consciousness. This information will help in diagnosing the cause of the seizure and deciding on the appropriate treatment. If seizures recur and no underlying causes can be identified, a person may suffer from epilepsy which, fortunately, can usually be controlled with medication.

SYMPTOMS

Strange sensations such as noises in the ears, flashes of light, nausea, dizziness, fear or anxiety can appear before an attack. Some sufferers recognize these and know when a seizure is about to occur. During a seizure, the casualty may:
- Black out or lose consciousness and fall.
- Exhibit confused behaviour.
- Cease breathing temporarily.
- Drool or froth at the mouth.
- Experience tingling or twitching in one part of the body.
- Experience vigorous muscle spasms causing the limbs to twitch and jerk.
- Grunt and snort.
- Lose bladder or bowel control.
- The head or eyes may move erratically.

CAUSES
- Intoxication/overdose (alcohol or drugs)
- Brain infection
- Injury to the brain or the head
- Choking
- Adverse effects of drugs
- Electric shock
- Epilepsy
- Fever (young children)
- High blood pressure (particularly during late pregnancy)
- Hypoglycaemia (low blood sugar)
- Heat Intolerance
- Poisoning
- Stroke

TREATMENT

- The first priority is to **prevent injury**. Clear away furniture or other objects that could cause harm.
- **Loosen tight clothing**, particularly around the casualty's neck, if possible.
- **If the casualty vomits**, turn the head to face downwards so vomited material is ejected from the mouth and not taken into the lungs.
- If you think a **high fever** could have caused a seizure in a young child, cool him gradually using cool compresses and tepid water.
- **Many people go into a deep sleep following a seizure**; cover them with a blanket to keep them warm, check that their airway, breathing and heartbeat are normal and let them to sleep. Do not be alarmed if they are disorientated after waking.
- If an unconscious casualty is **diabetic** or you think he may be, you can place some sugar granules or liquid glucose under the tongue. In the case of a casualty who has regained consciousness, it will be safe to provide some sugar water or concentrated liquid glucose. **Note:** Attempt this only once the seizure has ended, not while it is in progress.

PREVENTION

- If you have epilepsy, take your prescribed medication regularly and wear a Medic Alert tag (*see* p43) at all times.
- Treat high fevers (39°C+), especially in children.
- Ensure that chronic medications are taken as directed, particularly in children and the elderly.

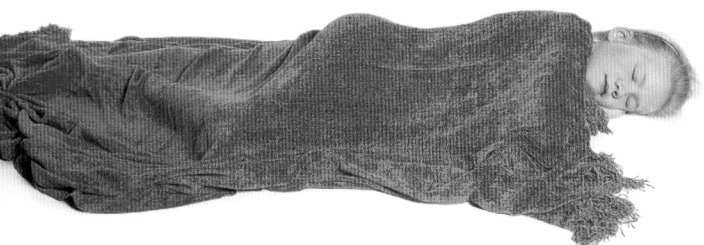

Cover the casualty with a light blanket as he/she is likely to sleep after a seizure.

SEEK MEDICAL HELP IF:

- the casualty has a seizure lasting longer than two minutes.
- he or she suffers more than one seizure in an hour.
- the casualty does not regain consciousness between successive seizures.
- there is absolutely no previous history of convulsions.
- the patient is a diabetic or suffers from high blood pressure.
- the casualty is pregnant.
- the seizure occurred in the water.

X DO NOT

- forcibly restrain the casualty; merely try to restrict the worst of the convulsions to prevent injury;
- place anything – handle of a spoon or your fingers – between the casualty's teeth during a seizure;
- move the casualty unless they are in danger or near something hazardous;
- try to stop the casualty convulsing;
- give rescue breaths to a seizure casualty, even if they are turning blue. Most seizures end well before brain damage can begin;
- give the casualty anything to eat or drink until the convulsions have stopped completely and you are satisfied that they are fully awake and alert.

Fever and meningitis

Fever is the body's response to illness and infection. Normal temperature is in the region of 37°C (98.6° F), with small variations from one individual to another. Temperature varies throughout the day, it is usually lower in the morning. Factors that influence temperature include stress, the amount of clothing worn, exercise, medication, age (children have a tendency to develop high fevers) and a woman's menstrual cycle. A low-grade fever is one of 38°C (100°F) or lower; high-grade fever is above 39°C (102°F). Most fevers are caused by infection. Fevers may peak suddenly and then subside, or come and go over a period of time. They may be accompanied by chills and shivering, as bacteria, viruses or toxins are released into the bloodstream.

 SEEK MEDICAL HELP IF:

- the fever remains above 39.5°C (103°F) after an hour or two of home treatment.
- the temperature rises above 40°C (105°F) at any time.
- the fever lasts two days or longer.
- the patient is a baby younger than six months of age.
- a child between six and 12 months has a fever for more than 24 hours.
- you think you may have taken or given the wrong medication or dosage.
- the patient develops a stiff neck, or becomes confused, irritable or sluggish.

CAUSES

- Colds or flu-like illnesses
- Ear infection, sore throat and 'strep' throat
- Upper respiratory tract infections (such as tonsillitis, pharyngitis, laryngitis)
- Acute bronchitis or pneumonia
- Viral or bacterial gastroenteritis
- Infections of the urinary tract (the bladder and the kidneys)
- Overdressing infants in hot weather or when a room is too warm

FEVER

Feverish patients send out mixed signals – the body temperature is raised, but the patient is shivering and suffers from chills. They are not cold, however, so do not cover them with blankets, you'll only raise the temperature higher. With a mild fever, all the patient needs is to rest and drink fluids. Other measures may include bathing in tepic water or sponging the patient down. Do not use cold water or rubbing alcohol as this can be easily absorbed through the skin. Some medications can be given to fight a fever or chills, but you should exercise caution. Aspirin should never be given to a child under the age of 12. If in doubt, do not provide any medication and summon medical attention.

REDUCING FEVER

Fever can be brought down by giving two paracetamol tablets to an adult (use the recommended dose of paracetamol syrup for children). Cool adult's fever by wiping the patient down with a cool, damp cloth, and give him or her plenty to drink.

If a child's temperature is still over 39.7°C (103.5°F) one to two hours after giving medication, remove their clothing, seat them in a bath of tepid water up to the navel and gently sponge their upper body, adding more warm water to the bath as necessary, to prevent shivering. The water must not be cold. When the fever is down, pat the child dry, put on light, loose garments, give it plenty of liquids and ensure that the room remains comfortably cool.

✗ DO NOT

- give aspirin to children under 12 and ibuprofen to infants under six months old.
- use iced water or rubbing alcohol to reduce a child's temperature.
- bundle a feverish child in blankets.
- wake a sleeping child to give it medication or check temperature. Sleep does more good than you realize.

MENINGITIS

This inflammation of the brain membranes can be caused by a virus or by bacteria. Viral meningitis, the most common form, is milder. Most cases of viral meningitis infections occur in children under the age of five. Acute bacterial meningitis must be treated as a medical emergency, as it can result in brain damage or death.

SYMPTOMS (MENINGITIS)

- Fever and chills, panting
- Severe headache
- Nausea and vomiting
- A stiff neck
- Pink-purple rash
- Sensitivity to light
- Loss of appetite
- Confusion or decreased consciousness
- Agitation, or irritability
- In babies it may look as though the fontanelles (*see* **glossary** p166) bulge out

The 'Glass Test'

If the child has developed a pinkish-purplish rash, press the side of a glass firmly against it. If it is just a rash, then the discolouration should fade and lose colour under pressure. If it does not change colour, however, and you can still see the rash clearly through the glass, contact your doctor immediately.

MENINGITIS TREATMENT

Seek medical care immediately. Speed is often the key to a successful outcome.

METHODS OF TEMPERATURE READING

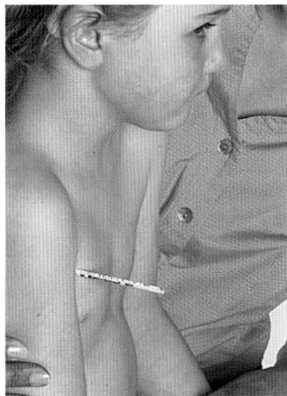
In the armpit

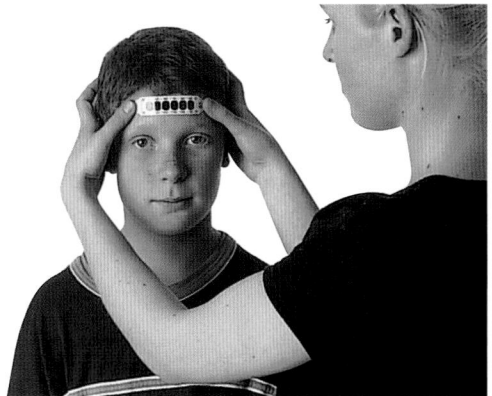
Strip against forehead

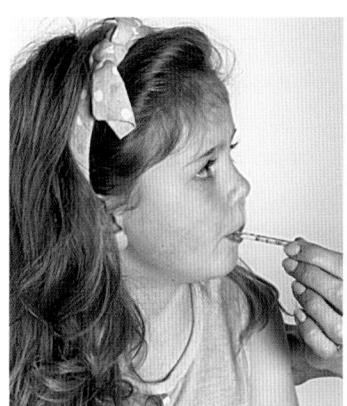
Under the tongue

Poisoning

If a person suddenly becomes ill for no apparent reason, consider whether they might have ingested or inhaled poison. Household products, plant matter, decaying food, pesticides, chemicals and narcotics can all result in poisoning. In addition, many medicines designed to be beneficial in small quantities, can be very dangerous when taken in excess.

Speed is absolutely crucial, so contact the nearest poison information centre or hotline, or your local emergency services, immediately you suspect poisoning. Look for containers from which the contents may have been consumed. The label should contain essential information which will be required by the doctors. Even if the label is partially destroyed, take the container along with you to the emergency room. Small children are particularly at risk, as they cannot distinguish poisonous substances from those that are not harmful, and they naturally put things into their mouths. Ensure that potentially dangerous items are, at all times, kept in locked cupboards or on high shelves.

SYMPTOMS

Affecting the stomach, appearance and general sense of wellness:
- Nausea and vomiting
- Abdominal pain
- Fever
- Headache
- Skin rash or burns
- Diarrhoea
- Loss of bladder control
- Irritability
- Loss of appetite
- Lips have bluish hue
- Unusual breath odour

Affecting breathing, circulation and the nervous system:
- Shortness of breath
- Dizziness
- Heart palpitations
- Chest pain
- Double vision
- Confusion
- Muscle twitching
- Drowsiness or stupor
- Numbness or tingling
- General feeling of weakness
- Seizures
- Unconsciousness

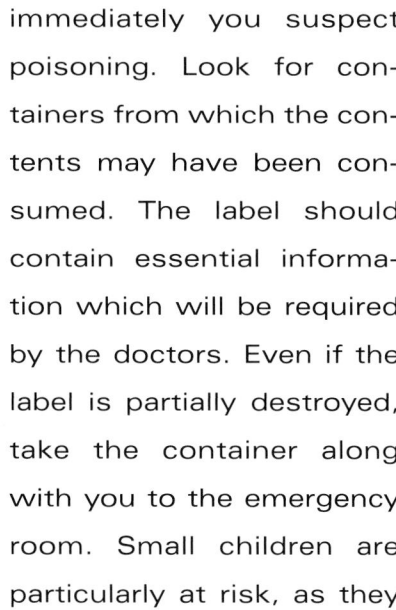

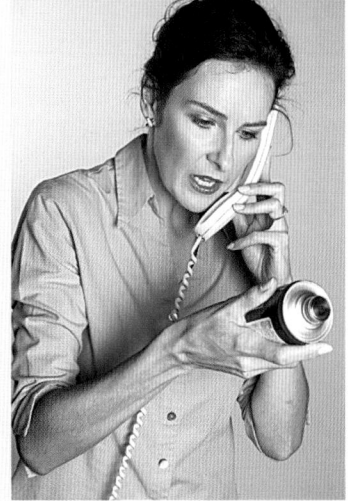

Above: In order to prescribe the correct treatment, your doctor will need to know the contents of the poisonous substance inhaled or consumed.

CAUSES

Ingested (swallowed):

- Food poisoning (such as botulism) caused by eating food that has become contaminated.
- Accidental or deliberate overdosing on medicines, either prescribed or over-the-counter.
- Eating poisonous plants. If you are not sure what the plant is, take a piece to the emergency room for identification
- Accidentally drinking solvents that were stored in cool-drink bottles.
- Overdosing on narcotic drugs, either by swallowing or injection.

Inhaled:

- The fumes or vapours from household cleaners or chemicals.
- Insecticides, pesticides or weedkillers can be inhaled while working in the garden.
- Carbon monoxide gas (from furnaces or motor vehicle exhausts).
- Abuse of solvents, adhesives and other substances to get 'high'.

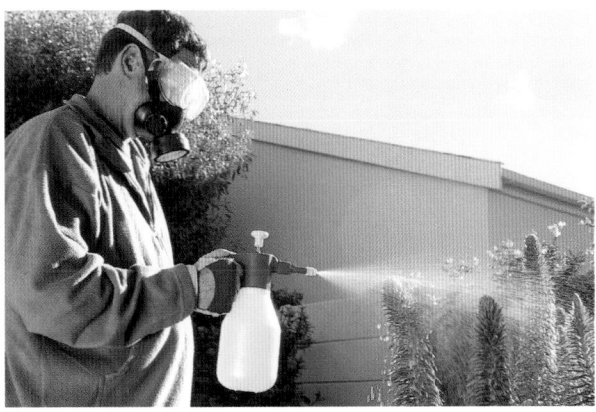

When spraying plants, wear a mask and goggles to prevent yourself from inhaling the chemicals.

Contact poisons:

- Exposure to household detergents, cleaners and chemicals.
- Exposure to toxins (venom) produced by some snakes and spiders.

TREATMENT

If the casualty is conscious and breathing normally, the first step is to contact your nearest doctor or emergency room. They will tell you what to do until help arrives. Ask the casualty what they ingested or inhaled. If they are unable to give a coherent reply, look for anything that may give a clue, such as empty containers. Try to ascertain the type of poisoning by checking for burns around the mouth, unusual breath odours, vomiting or laboured breathing.

Ingested (swallowed) poison:

- If the casualty is unconscious and not breathing, check the **vital signs** (*see* p165) and begin **rescue breaths** (*see* p26) and **chest compressions** (*see* pp22–27). Monitor until medical help arrives. While waiting and as soon as casualty is breathing unaided, place them in the **recovery position** (*see* p25) and keep calm and comfortable.
- Never induce vomiting (unless told to do so by the poison control centre).
- If the casualty vomits, clear the airway (use one finger wrapped in a cloth). Save as much of the vomitus as you can in a container. If the casualty ate part of a plant, fragments in the material will aid identification, and the same goes for pills that might have been consumed.
- If **convulsions** (*see* p44) begin, protect the casualty from injury and give appropriate first aid.
- Clothing soaked in a chemical or toxic substance should be removed and the affected body area washed with water. For poison in dry powder form, brush off (away from the face) as much as you can, remove clothing and wash the affected area.

Inhaled poison:

- The first step is to remove the person and yourself from the source of the poison. If you are uncertain of the source, or you suspect fumes are still present, try to have someone else on stand-by, in case you also succumb.
- Take deep breaths of fresh air, hold your breath, cover your mouth and nose with a wet cloth and drag the casualty into the open air. If you cannot do that, open doors and windows, or use a fan.

- Once out of the danger area, check the casualty's **vital signs** (*see* pp22–3 and p165). Begin **rescue breaths** (*see* p26) and/or **chest compressions** (*see* pp22–27) if required.
- An inhaled poison, such as an insecticide, might have affected the eyes or skin. Check these and administer the appropriate first aid (*see* **eye injuries** p62).
- If the casualty vomits or convulses, treat as indicated above.

PREVENTION

The average home contains many substances that can be highly dangerous when taken or used incorrectly. One of the easiest ways to prevent accidental poisoning at home is to educate your children, as soon as they are old enough, not to touch any substances that have not been approved by you.

In the home

- Keep all medicines, household cleaners, garden products, and solvents locked away, and keep the keys kept out of reach of children.
- Never use food or soft-drink containers to store anything other than food or drinks.
- Keep hazardous substances in their original containers. If a container starts leaking, transfer the contents to a new non-food/drink container and label it clearly. If possible, remove the old label, or photocopy it and use it to identify the new container. Transfer safety warnings as well.

- Always wash fruits and vegetables thoroughly before use.
- Prepare and cook food in hygienic conditions and discard any items that might have gone off or be contaminated in some way.
- Be aware of food allergies. Someone allergic to peanuts, for instance, can develop breathing difficulties if nut products are used in a dish (*see* **anaphylactic shock** p42).
- Check food when purchasing to ensure the 'sell by' date has not been reached.

DO NOT

- give an unconscious casualty anything by mouth.
- induce vomiting unless instructed to do so by medical personnel (any poison that burned on the way down will do so again on the way up and increase the damage).
- try to neutralize the poison, unless told to do so by a medical expert.
- give any emetics (such as Ipecac).

In the garden

- Remove toxic plants from your garden.
- Never eat wild berries, mushrooms or any other plants unless you are absolutely certain that they are safe.
- When using insecticides or garden sprays, remember that even a light breeze could blow the mist back onto your face or body, or through an open window into the house. If the kitchen windows are open, food could easily be contaminated.
- Keep pets out of the way when you are working with garden sprays and other chemicals.

CARBON MONOXIDE POISONING

Carbon monoxide is a colourless, odourless gas. It is produced during combustion in vehicle engines, charcoal-burning barbecues, portable propane heaters, or portable or non-ventilated natural gas appliances such as a shower-head water heater. Under normal circumstances, when you inhale, you take in air containing oxygen. Carbon monoxide interferes with the blood's ability to carry oxygen, thereby progressively starving the tissues of oxygen, leading to the symptoms mentioned below.

SYMPTOMS

- Headache
- Nausea and vomiting
- Impaired judgement
- Hyperactivity
- Irritability
- Abnormal or rapid heart beat
- Rapid breathing
- Shortness of breath
- Low blood pressure
- Fainting
- Chest pain
- Convulsions
- Coma, followed by unconsciousness and death

CAUSES

Carbon monoxide poisoning occurs in confined or non-ventilated spaces, so be careful when using any appliance that involves combustion in its operation.

Carbon monoxide poisoning may occur accidentally, by working on a vehicle engine and keeping the garage door closed in cold weather, for example; or deliberately, by running the engine in the same conditions in order to commit suicide.

Because you cannot smell carbon monoxide, poisoning can occur more easily than if you could detect its presence.

TREATMENT

Get the casualty into fresh air, as this will immediately halt the level of contamination. If the carbon monoxide levels are very high, you could be in danger yourself, particularly if breathing hard from anxiety or exertion.

- Take three deep breaths, hold your breath, enter the area and get the casualty out into fresh air. Drag them out by their clothing, legs or whatever, if this will reduce your exposure. Leave the door open to ventilate the area.
- Call for medical assistance immediately. If possible, inform the dispatcher of the casualty's condition, age, weight and the length of time they have been exposed to the carbon monoxide.
- If the casualty has ceased breathing and there is no pulse, administer **resuscitation** (*see* pp22–37) while awaiting the arrival of medical assistance.
- Recovery is usually slow and, depending on the severity of the attack, there may be permanent brain damage with impaired mental ability. If the latter is still apparent after two weeks, complete recovery is not very likely. Even though the victim may seem free of symptoms, impaired mental ability can appear within a week or two of the incident.

PREVENTION

Install carbon monoxide detectors in areas in which gas appliances are used, such as the kitchen, bathroom, garage and workshop.

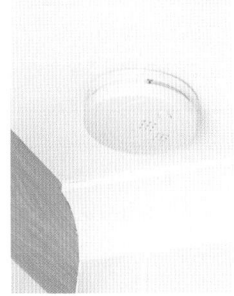

Carbon monoxide detector.

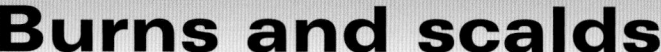

Burns and scalds

Burns are among the most common injuries, although fortunately, the vast majority are comparatively minor. They are graded in severity (see box). Providing the appropriate first aid can reduce the consequences of a burn injury but medical attention is vital if the burn is serious (second- or third-degree), does not heal properly, or complications, such as infection, set in afterwards. When in doubt as to a burn's severity, always treat it as serious. Be particularly alert if the burn is not painful – this could mean a severe burn in which the nerves have been destroyed. (*See* p53 for information on **treating minor burns and scalds**.)

SYMPTOMS

Airway burns:
- Burns on the head, neck or face, including a charred mouth and/or burned lips
- Coughing and wheezing
- Carbon-stained mucus or saliva
- Laboured, difficult breathing
- Singed nose hairs or eyebrows
- Voice change

(Note: Severe airway burns can occur in the absence of any surface burn, for example, if a person is caught in a smoke-filled room.)

Surface burns:
- Blisters
- Pain (in the absence of pain, suspect a severe burn)
- Peeling skin
- Red skin
- White or charred skin
- Swelling around the affected area
- **Shock** (*see* p40) – signs include pale, clammy skin, bluish lips and fingernails, weakness, disorientation and decreasing alertness

A NUMBER OF FACTORS DETERMINE THE SEVERITY OF A BURN

- **Size** – the extent of the body covered.
- **Locality** – burns on face, hands, feet and genitalia tend to be more serious because of possible loss of function, either while the burn heals, or permanently.
- **Degree and type of heat** (i.e. flame, electricity, or hot oil). Burns from a chemical or toxic substance may result in other complications.
- **Length of time** the casualty was exposed to the heat source (brief or prolonged exposure).
- **Age** – children under four and adults over 60 years old tend to develop complications more readily than other age groups.

CAUSES

- Thermal burns are caused by dry, radiated heat such as from a fire, hot surface (heaters or stoves), or the sun.
- Scalding is caused by hot liquid or steam.
- Chemical burns come from skin contact with chemicals, including some household products.
- Electrical burns result from contact with a live wire or current.
- Friction burns are common in sports injuries or motorcycle accidents.
- Smoke, super-heated air or toxic fumes can cause burn injuries to the airways.

TREATMENT OF MINOR BURNS AND SCALDS

The prime objective is to reduce the heat that still remains in the tissue.

- **Remove the source of heat**.
- **Reassure the casualty**.
- **Remove watches and rings** as well as other restricting items before swelling begins.
- **If the skin is intact**, gently run cool (not ice-cold) water over the burn area or soak in a basin of cool water for at least 10 minutes.
- **Once the burn area has been cooled, cover it with a clean cloth or sterile bandage**. Try not to subject the burn to friction and do not tie the dressing too tightly.
- If necessary **use a mild over-the-counter pain medication to reduce the pain**. Minor burns do not usually require further treatment, other than a change of dressing.

A minor burn or scald can be soothed by holding it under cool running water before it is loosely bandaged in sterile dressing, or cling wrap to avoid infection of the affected area.

TREATMENT OF MAJOR BURNS AND SCALDS

Always treat these as serious and call for immediate medical assistance.

- **Remove the casualty from the heat source**, so if someone's clothing is on fire, pour water over them or hose them down (use a gentle spray).
- If water is not available, wrap the casualty in a thick coat or blanket made of natural fibres, such as cotton or wool, to **smother the flames**. (Do not use items made of synthetic fibre, such as nylon, as they could ignite).
- Lay the casualty flat and roll him on the ground.
- **Ensure all smouldering or burning garments are fully extinguished**.
- **Do not remove items of burnt clothing unless they come off easily**.
- **Ensure the casualty is breathing** before attending to the burn. If the airway is blocked, open it. If breathing does not restart spontaneously, begin **rescue breaths** (*see* p26).
- **Place a cool, moist, sterile bandage, or kitchen clingfilm (pvc wrap) over the burn area**. Do not use a blanket or towel as fibres may get into the burn and cause complications later.
- If fingers, feet or inner surfaces of the legs have been burned, **keep injured surfaces separated** with dry, sterile, non-adhesive dressings. A pillow slip or plastic shopping bag can be tied around burnt hands or feet.
- **Raise the burn area**, protecting it from being subjected to pressure and friction.
- **Prevent shock** by lying the casualty down and raising their feet about 30cm (12in) unless a head, neck or back injury is suspected. Keep them warm by covering with a coat or blanket.
- **Monitor the casualty's vital signs** until medical help arrives.

TYPES OF BURNS

- **First-degree** (superficial) – minor burns to the outer skin layer look like mild to moderate sunburn (reddish, hot skin).
- **Second-degree** (partial thickness) – deeper burns that damage both the outer and underlying skin layers result in pain, redness, swelling and blistering. If precautions are not taken, blisters can become infected.
- **Third-degree** (full thickness) – serious burns affecting both outer and underlying skin layers, causing extreme pain, redness, swelling and blistering. Third-degree burns extend into deep tissues, causing brown or blackened skin that may be numb.

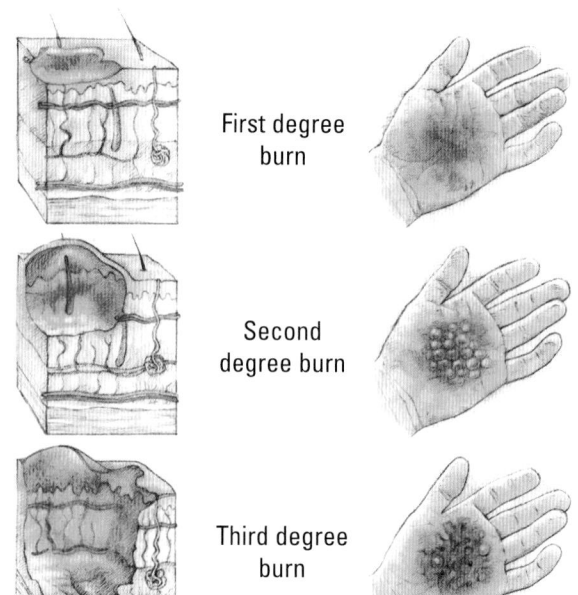

First degree burn

Second degree burn

Third degree burn

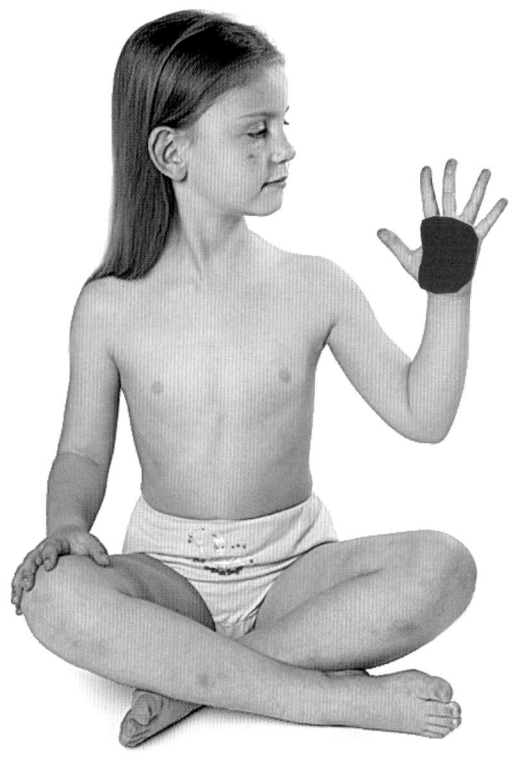

⚠ CAUTION

Call for emergency medical assistance if:
- a burn is large, severe or there is any difficulty with breathing.
- any burn affects the face, hands or groin.
- a child under two years of age is burnt.
- it is a chemical or electrical burn.
- the casualty shows signs of **shock** (*see* p40).
- treat a second-degree burn as a major burn if it is greater than 50–75mm (2–3in) in diameter, or is on the hands, feet, face, groin, buttocks, or a major joint.

The surface area of a burn may be estimated using the hand as a measure. The palm is equivalent to 1% of Total Body Surface Area (TBSA). As a rule, any burn involving more than 1% TBSA requires medical attention.

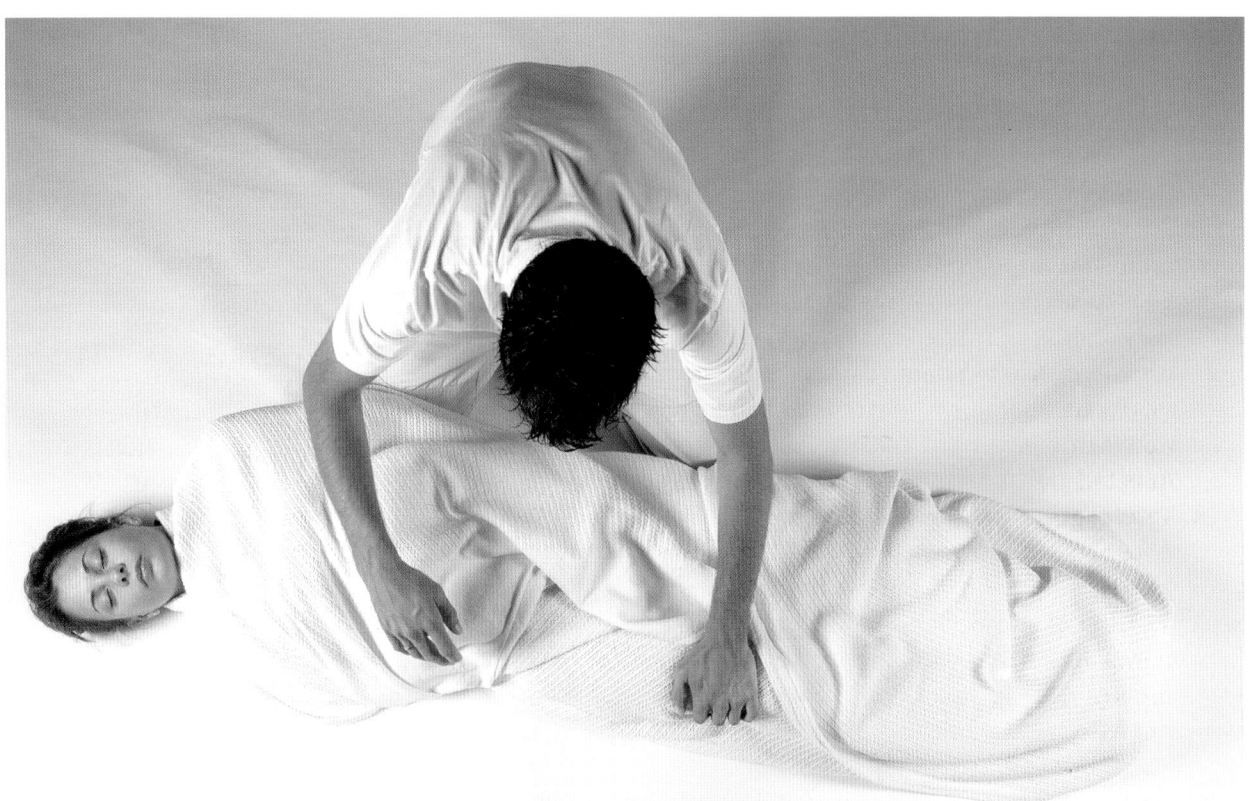

If clothing catches fire, roll the person up in a blanket made of natural fibre, such as cotton or wool, to smother the flames.

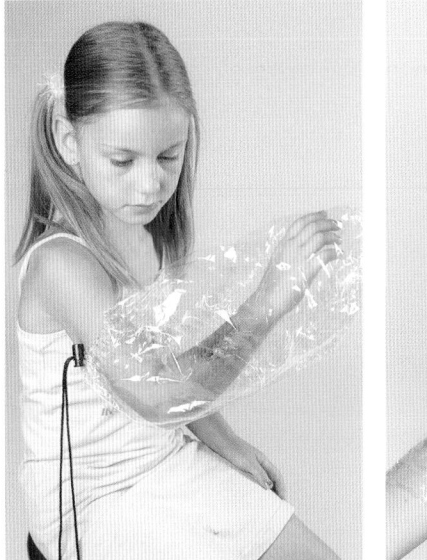
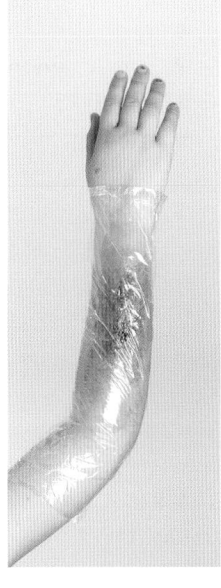

To prevent infection, loosely cover a severe burn with a clean plastic bag or cling wrap.

 DO NOT

- apply an adhesive bandage, cotton wool or fluffy cotton dressing, ice, medication, oil, ointment or any household remedy to a burn, as they can prevent proper healing, and possibly cause an infection.
- apply cold compresses or immerse a severe burn in cold water; this can cause reduced circulation and delay healing.
- breathe or cough on the burn.
- burst or puncture a blister.
- disturb or attempt to remove blistered or dead skin.
- give a severely burnt casualty anything by mouth.
- place a pillow under the casualty's head if there is an airway burn and he or she is lying down. This can restrict the airway.

PREVENTING BURN INJURIES

The easiest way to avoid being burned is to not go near hot things, but this is rarely possible in the normal course of daily living. Ovens and stoves, heaters and radiators, open fires and a host of small appliances are things we take for granted, and cannot imagine living without. While adults usually get burnt out of carelessness, children tend to burn themselves because they are ignorant of the dangers involved. It is every parent's duty to try and keep their children out of harm's way, by removing or reducing the potential for accidents or injuries to occur.

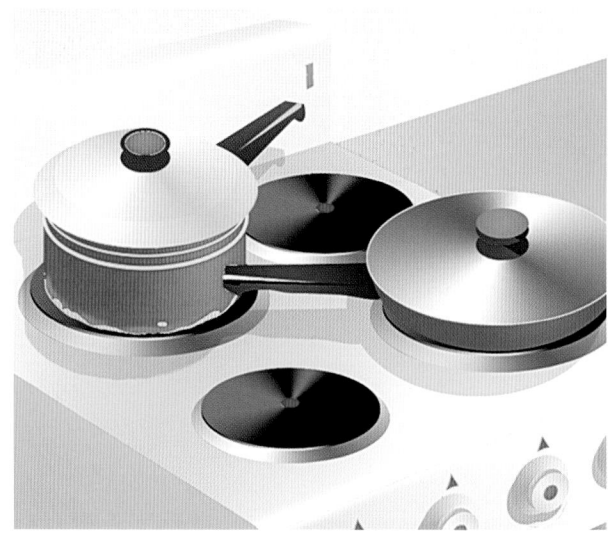

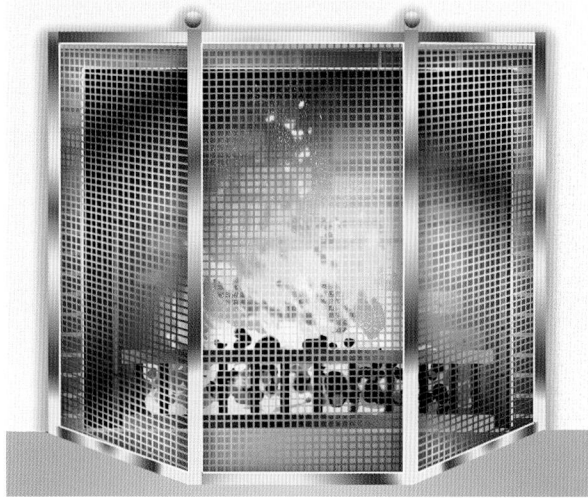

Install fireguards around open wood, coal or gas fires. Do not hang clothing or anything else on the fireguard – this only creates a hazard.

KITCHEN

More domestic fires start in the kitchen than anywhere else, making it the room with the greatest potential for burn-related accidents.

- Never leave anything unattended on the stove or under the grill. If you leave the kitchen, turn off the heat and/or move the pot to a cold plate.
- Use your oven timer to remind you when something needs to be removed from the oven.
- Make sure your oven gloves and pot holders are in good condition. It is easy to burn your hands if there are holes or gaps in the fabric.

- Turn pot handles away from the edge of a stove or countertop and make use of the back plates.
- When lifting the lid off a boiling pot, don't bend over it, or you could scald your face as the steam escapes.
- Watch your hands when doing the ironing, a lapse in concentration can result in burnt fingers.

BATHROOM

A child left in the bath unattended could turn on the hot tap and suffer severe **burns** (*see* p52) in a very short space of time.

BEDROOM

Electric blankets account for thousands of fires every year. Don't use a blanket that has worn or frayed wiring, or shows signs of scorching. Ensure plug and control connections are secure and don't leave it switched on for hours. Turn the blanket off when you get into/out of bed. Consider replacing electric blankets that are more than 10 years old.

OUTDOORS

Summer is barbecue time, which means flames, hot coals and the potential for burns. Prevent children from playing around the cooking area, keep some water on hand to douse any flare-ups and dispose of hot coals safely, not where some little foot could stand on them.

Chemical burns and injuries

Most chemical burns are the result of accidental contact with an abrasive substance. The inadvertent ingestion of such a substance (*see* **poisoning** p48) can cause severe internal damage. The degree of injury depends on the amount of chemical involved, where on (or in) the body it landed and the length of time the casualty was exposed to it. Certain chemicals, including battery acid, common household bleach and swimming-pool acid, can cause problems ranging from relatively mild effects (including burns), to much more serious reactions. Immediately suspect exposure to a chemical if an otherwise healthy person (or pet) becomes ill for no apparent reason. See whether you can find a chemical container nearby.

SYMPTOMS

These vary, depending on the chemical to which the casualty was exposed, and the amount and duration of the exposure.

Chemical poisoning:
- Abdominal pain
- Breathing difficulty
- Convulsions (seizures)
- Dizziness
- Headache
- Hives, itching, swelling
- Nausea or vomiting
- Weakness resulting from an allergic reaction
- Unconsciousness

Burns:
- Bright red or bluish rash on the skin and lips
- Pain where the skin has made contact with a toxic substance
- Blisters, burns on the skin

CAUSES

- Chemical burns are caused by accidental skin contact with a toxic or corrosive substance.
- Poisoning results from either the ingestion of too much medicine or taking the wrong medication (accidental overdose), or from deliberately swallowing medicines or chemical substances, as in a suicide attempt.

TIP

If possible, keep the chemical container and hand it to the paramedic or doctor. The information on the container will assist the medical personnel with an approproate diagnosis and suitable treatment.

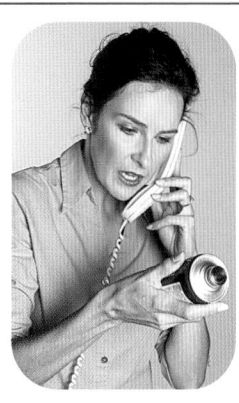

TREATMENT

Minor surface chemical burns will generally heal without further treatment. However, if there are second- or third-degree **burns** (*see* p54), call for medical assistance immediately. Medical help should also be obtained without delay in the case of a chemical being ingested.

- If possible, **remove deposits of the chemical from clothes or skin**, doing your utmost to avoid contact. If the chemical is dry, brush it off. If there is a breeze, brush away from the eyes and downwind, covering the casualty's eyes and protecting your own to avoid contamination. If a chemical does get into the eyes, flush them with water for at least 15 minutes and call for medical help.
- R**emove contaminated clothing**, including jewellery (a watch or ring, for instance, could trap deposits of the chemical).
- **Flush away any remaining chemical residue on the body**, using cool running water for at least 15 minutes. (*See* below.)

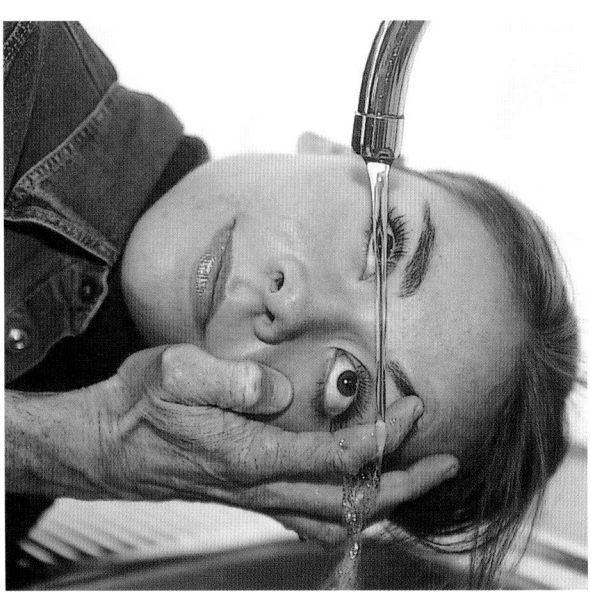

- Treat the casualty for **shock** (*see* p40) if they appear faint or pale, or if their breathing sounds shallow or rapid.
- Apply cool, wet compresses to relieve pain.

- **Dry the burn and cover it with a dry sterile dressing or clean cloth**. Protect the burn from pressure and friction.
- **Watch carefully for systemic reactions** and treat the casualty accordingly while awaiting medical assistance.

PREVENTION

- Toxic products are found in many household products and incorrect use can be dangerous. Always follow the manufacturer's instructions and observe any precautions.
- Keep exposure to chemicals to a minimum – over time, even low-level contamination can cause health problems.
- Select products that are contained in child-proof, secure containers, keep them in those containers and with labels intact.
- Keep chemicals away from food, children and pets, as well as kitchen surfaces.
- Re-seal the container immediately after use and store securely in a lockable cupboard or on a high shelf, out of the reach of toddlers.
- Never mix chemicals – the result could be dangerous. The concoction might produce harmful fumes, or even explode.
- Always handle substances that produce fumes (such as paints, solvents and ammonia) in well-ventilated areas.
- Never put chemicals (solvents for example) into cool-drink bottles or food containers.

X DO NOT

- allow the chemical to contaminate you as you give first aid.
- try to neutralize a chemical without getting medical advice from your nearest poison control centre or doctor.
- disturb a blister or remove dead skin.
- apply any ointment or salve.

Head injuries

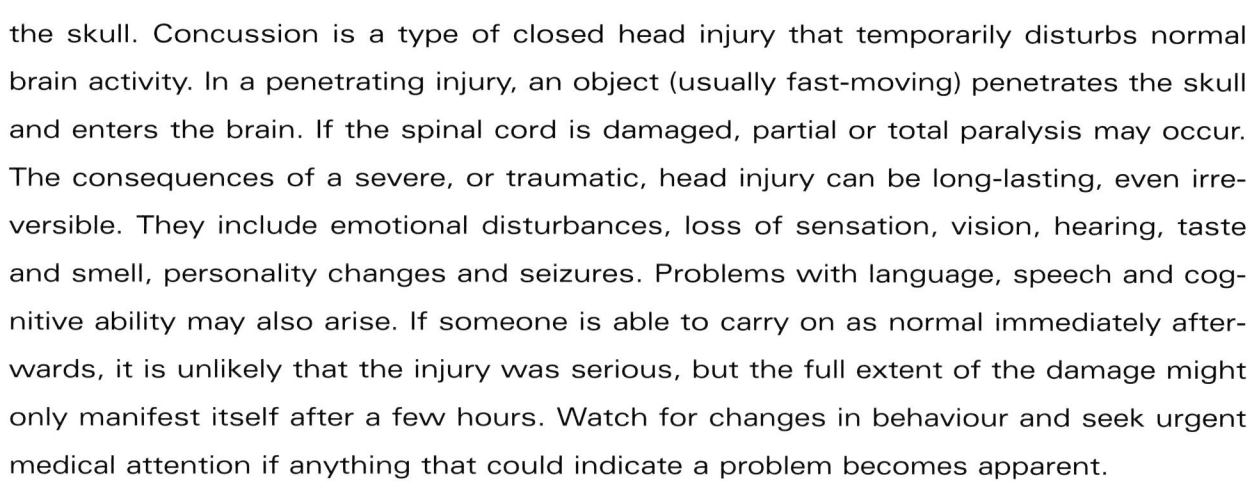

Head injuries are classified as either closed or penetrating. In a closed injury, usually caused by a blow to the head or due to the head hitting a solid surface, the force does not penetrate the skull. Concussion is a type of closed head injury that temporarily disturbs normal brain activity. In a penetrating injury, an object (usually fast-moving) penetrates the skull and enters the brain. If the spinal cord is damaged, partial or total paralysis may occur. The consequences of a severe, or traumatic, head injury can be long-lasting, even irreversible. They include emotional disturbances, loss of sensation, vision, hearing, taste and smell, personality changes and seizures. Problems with language, speech and cognitive ability may also arise. If someone is able to carry on as normal immediately afterwards, it is unlikely that the injury was serious, but the full extent of the damage might only manifest itself after a few hours. Watch for changes in behaviour and seek urgent medical attention if anything that could indicate a problem becomes apparent.

SYMPTOMS

Not all head injuries are cause for concern. The list below is intended to assist you in diagnosing the seriousness of the injury yourself before medical help arrives:

Scalp
- bruising at the site of impact
- a small cut at the site of impact

Skull
- accumulation of blood under the scalp soon after the accident could indicate a skull fracture
- headache
- clear or blood-stained fluid leaking from the nose or ears

Neck
- pain or stiffness in the neck
- a feeling of weakness, or pins-and-needles sensations in the arms or legs could indicate injury to the spinal cord
- severe neck injury may be accompanied by breathing difficulties (resulting from paralysis of the diaphragm and chest muscles)

Brain
- *mild concussion* is indicated by headache, irritability, nausea and vomiting (especially in children)
- *severe concussion* is indicated by a temporary loss of consciousness. Convulsions (fits) are possible, as is nausea

CAUSES

One of the most common causes of head injuries is vehicle accidents, and children are particularly vulnerable if they are not suitably restrained in safety seats. Accidental blows to the head, or falls sustained during sports and other recreational activities also common causes of head injuries.

TREATMENT

In the case of a minor bump on the head, observe the person for a few hours (checking their level of consciousness, heart rate and respiratory rate regularly). If no symptoms develop, the injury was mild and no treatment is required other than a painkiller or cold compress.

If the casualty exhibits any of the following symptoms, summon immediate medical assistance without delay:

- **If the casualty is unconscious** but their breathing and pulse is satisfactory, treat as for a **spinal injury** (*see* pp74–5). Stabilize the neck by placing both hands on either side of the head and keep it in that position until help arrives.
- **Stem scalp bleeding** by firmly pressing a clean cloth on the wound, without moving the casualty's head. Place a second cloth over the first if the latter becomes soaked.
- **Do not apply direct pressure** to an injury if you think the skull may be fractured.

- **Do not remove any debris** from a wound. Cover it with a sterile gauze dressing and wait for medical help to arrive.
- Apply ice packs to bruises under the scalp.
- If the casualty is vomiting, do not turn the head (in case there is a spinal injury). Instead, roll the head and body as one, supporting the head and neck in the same relative position to the body, to

✗ DO NOT

- move the casualty unless necessary.
- shake a dazed casualty in an attempt to get a response.
- pick up a fallen child when there is any sign of a head injury.
- remove any object sticking out of a head wound.
- remove a motor cyclist's helmet if you suspect a head injury (unless breathing is compromised). This really needs two people to execute, otherwise you could aggravate a neck injury.
- wash a head wound that is very deep or bleeding profusely.
- consume alcohol within 48 hours after suffering a head injury.

CAUTION

- In the case of serious head injury, you should always assume that the cervical spinal cord has been injured. Ensure that the casualty's head and neck are well stabilized and well protected until medical help arrives.

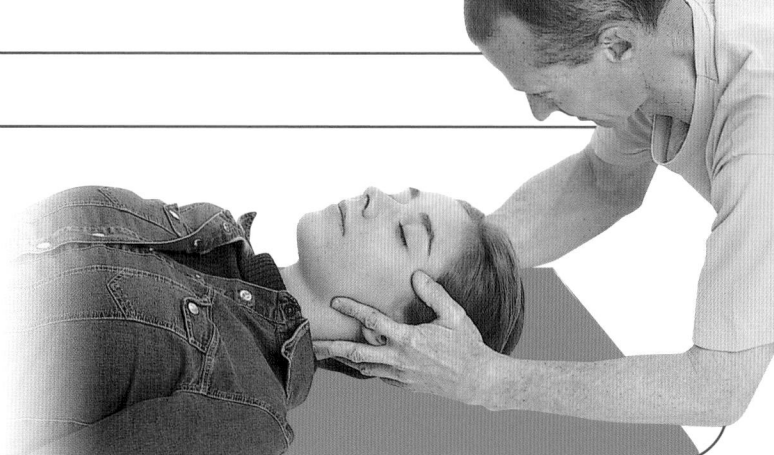

prevent choking. Children often vomit once after sustaining a minor head injury, but if there is repeated vomiting, or if the child becomes drowsy, contact a doctor.

In all of the above instances, the sooner help arrives the better. While you wait, check the vital signs (*see* p165) and begin **rescue breaths** (*see* p26) and/or **chest compressions** (*see* p27).

PREVENTION

- Wear the correct seat belts when in a vehicle.
- Reduce your risk by not drinking and driving or allowing yourself to be driven by someone you suspect is drunk.
- Wear protective headgear when riding a bicycle, motorcycle or horse, or when mountain climbing, and an approved hard hat on construction sites.
- Ensure your child's play area is safe, and supervise them at play.
- If walking or jogging after dark, wear light-coloured clothing to make yourself more visible.

SKULL FRACTURE

If the skull undergoes severe trauma it can fracture, leading to possible brain injury, which can only be confirmed by an X-ray or brain scan. Fractures take a variety of forms:

- Simple – a break in the skull; no skin damage.
- Linear – a break resembling a thin line, with no splintering, depression, or distortion of the skull.
- Depressed – a 'crushed' portion of the skull, resembling a dent, is depressed inwards.
- Compound – a splintered fracture where the skull bones are broken at the site of the trauma.

FRACTURES OF THE JAW

It takes a lot of force to fracture the upper or lower jaw. However, you should suspect this injury if:

- you notice marked swelling or bruising of the gums, in the floor of the mouth or around the lower half of the face.
- the casualty is unable to open or close the mouth normally.
- you notice that the upper and lower sets of teeth

do not meet each other normally.
- two or more teeth appear displaced.

TREATMENT

- Ensure that the airway remains open by letting the casualty lean forward so that blood can drain from the mouth. Loose teeth can be kept and given to the doctor or emergency service.
- Let the casualty support the injured jaw by gently holding a soft cloth against it.
- Ensure that you get the casualty to a doctor or to a hospital as soon as possible.

INJURIES TO THE NOSE

A blow to the nose will often cause no more than a little swelling and some bleeding from one or both nostrils. Fractures of the nasal bones are usually caused by assault and will result in severe bruising and heavier bleeding. The fracture can only be confirmed with special X-rays of the face. The 'bones' of a child's nose are mostly soft, pliable cartilage until they begin to harden with calcium in the early teens, so true fractures of the nose are uncommon in young children. If you suspect a broken nose:

- Control the bleeding (*see* p38).
- Control bruising/swelling with a cold compress.
- Use a mild painkiller if necessary.

Seek a medical opinion when:

- the nose appears crooked after the swelling has gone down.
- there is persistent or recurrent bleeding from one or both nostrils.
- the casualty seems to have difficulty breathing through either nostril.
- the outer edge of the nostril has been lacerated.

TREATMENT

- Treat the bleeding nose (see pp88-9).
- Reduce the swelling by holding a cold, wet cloth loosely against the nose.
- If you suspect a more serious injury or fracture. ensure that you get the casualty to hopsital or to a doctor as soon as possible.

Eye injuries

Loss of sight can affect just about every aspect of your life, so treat as an emergency anything which could lead to loss of vision if left untreated – this includes ridding the eye of a foreign object but then experiencing persistent discomfort or pain. Have it checked!

Eye injuries can be caused by airborne objects, and can include cuts, scratches, burns, or a blow to the eye. Chemical injuries result from direct exposure when droplets splash into the eyes, or from fumes given off by household cleansers, pesticides, weedkillers, solvents, acids, alkaline substances and more. The workshop is particularly dangerous, as particles can fly into the eye at speed, either penetrating it or severely damaging its delicate surface. Sports injuries or fights can leave one with a black eye, when bleeding under the skin causes bruising or a dark discolouration of the surrounding area. This will disappear with time, but eye injuries should always be checked by your doctor.

SYMPTOMS

- Bleeding or bruising in or around the eye
- Double vision, or loss of vision
- Itching, stinging or burning eyes
- Pupils of unequal size
- Redness (bloodshot eyes)
- Scratchy feeling in the eye
- Sensitivity to light

TIP

Over-the-counter (OTC) eye drops contain mild vaso-constrictors (decongestants) and should only be used in the case of mild allergies or eye irritations. They should never be used to treat an injury or when there is any chance of an eye infection.

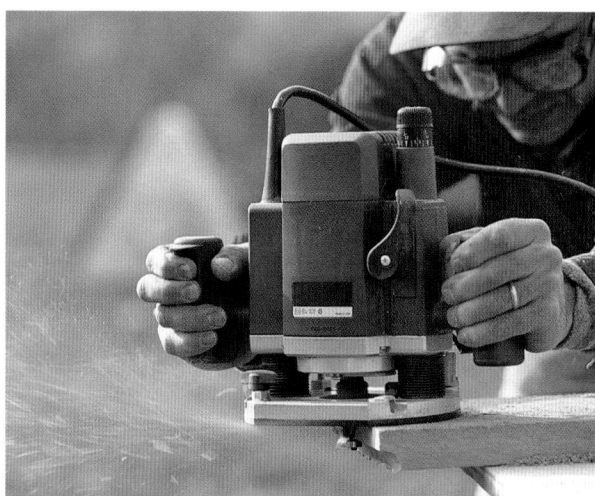

Protect your eyes by wearing plastic goggles whenever you are working with power tools, to prevent sawdust or metal shavings from shooting up into your eye. A foreign body in the eye can cause unpleasant irritation, and in some cases lasting damage. If you do get something in your eye, rinse with water immediately. If the irritation persists, see a doctor.

CAUSES
- Blow to the eye socket
- Foreign object in the eye
- Injury to the eyeball itself
- Chemical injury
- Medical conditions (i.e. infection or glaucoma)

TREATMENT
Object on the surface of the eye:
- If blinking or shedding tears do not expel the object, go to a well-illuminated area and check the eye as the casualty swivels their eyes from left to right and up and down until you spot the offending object.
- If you don't spot the object, gently pull the lower lid out and down to expose the fold between the eyelid and the globe of the eye. You may need to do the same to the upper lid.
- Once you spot the object, gently wash it out with water or a damp cotton-tipped swab; use the latter as a last resort and keep it away from the pupil.
- Do not try to remove an object embedded in the eyeball. Make an eye cup out of the bottom half of a styrofoam cup and secure this over the eye with strapping or plaster (*see picture at right*) to avoid aggravating the injury or inflammation.
- If you cannot find or remove the object, and the casualty still has discomfort or blurred vision, cover the eye and seek medical help.

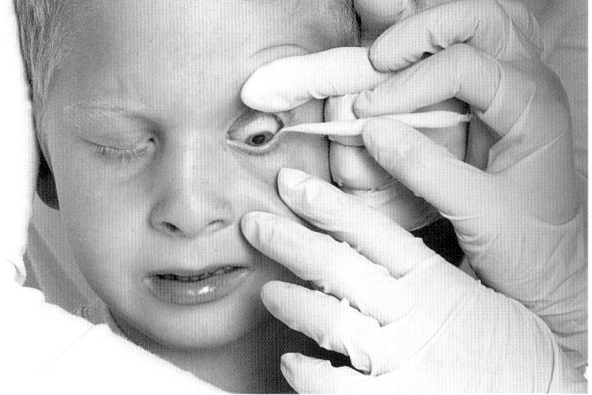

To remove a foreign body, moisten a clean cotton bud or piece of cotton wool. Lift the lid up and get the child to look down.

Object embedded in the eye:
- Do not apply any pressure to the object or try to remove it, and stop the casualty from rubbing or touching the eye.
- If the object is large, cut out the base of a paper or foam cup and place the cup over the injured eye, taping it into position (*see picture below*). If the object is small, cover both eyes with a clean cloth or sterile dressing to discourage eye movement.
- Keep the casualty quiet, calm and reassured until medical assistance is available.

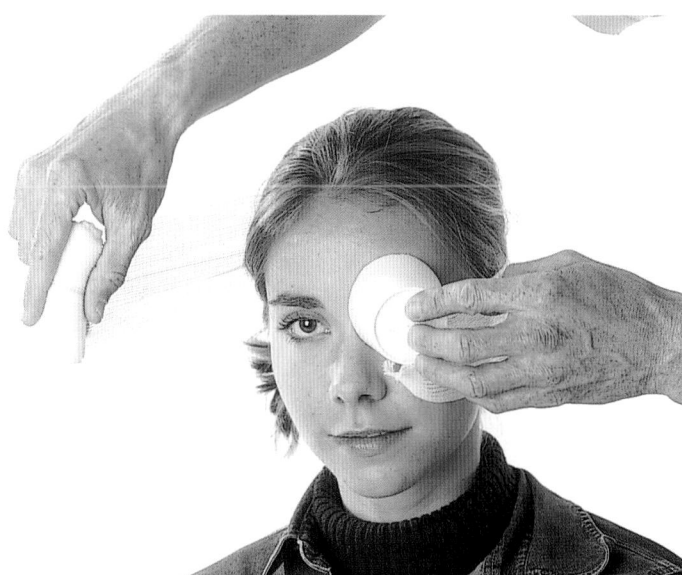

Bandage a paper cup in place to protect an injured eye until medical help can be obtained.

Chemical injury to the eye:
- Irrigate the eye immediately with tap water. Turn the casualty's head so the injured eye is down and to the side, hold the eyelid open, and run water in and over the eye for at least 20 minutes or until you have medical help.
- If the chemical has got into both eyes, get the casualty into the shower and hold their eyes open-

with their head tilted back. Do not run the shower full-blast as powerful droplets of water could add to the discomfort.

- Remove contact lenses, only after the eyes have been rinsed.
- Cover both eyes with a clean dressing and avoid rubbing the eyes.
- Get medical help urgently.

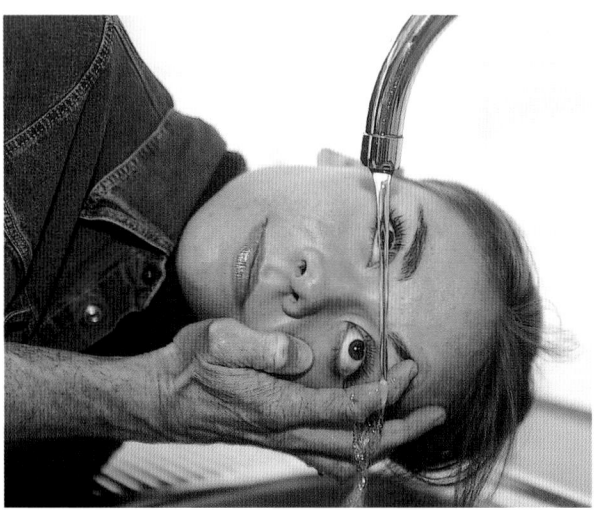

In the case of a chemical injury, wash the eye with cold water for at least 20 minutes.

Burns

- Gently pour cool water over and into the eyes (unless it is painful to do so) to reduce swelling and relieve the pain.
- Apply a cool compress to the eyes, but avoid applying pressure.
- If there is swelling in or around the eyes, if the lashes or lid skin is burned, or if there is any change in vision, seek medical help.

Cuts, scratches and blows to the eye

- Seek medical assistance immediately if the eyeball has been injured.
- Do not apply pressure to the eye.
- Gently apply cold compresses to reduce swelling and help stop bleeding, but do not apply pressure to control bleeding.

- If blood is pooling in the eye, cover both eyes with a clean cloth or sterile dressing to reduce eye movement. Get medical help immediately.
- Small cuts to the eyelid (less than a few millimetres long) should require little more than cleaning and dressing. However, if the eye can't be closed, or the cut is larger or deeper, or goes over the edge of the lid, cover the eye with a sterile pad and seek medical attention.

Double vision (diplopia)

This is a very serious symptom following an eye injury, as it may result from the displacement of the eyeball and traction on the delicate optic nerve. If a casualty complains of 'seeing double', seek urgent medical attention.

Stye

An infection of tiny glands situated on the lower edge of the upper and lower eyelid, causing very localized pain and redness of the lid. Styes usually disappear spontaneously, but see a doctor if pain persists.

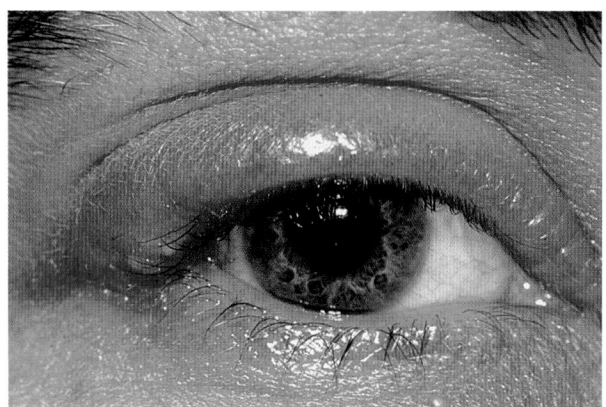

A stye is caused by inflammation of one of the hair follicles from which eyelashes grow. The condition, while not very serious, is unpleasant and unsightly. The eye itches and the movement of the eye lid causes discomfort. Cool the inflamed lid with a cold cloth and visit your doctor. The treatment is relatively quick and effective and may include a salve and eye drops.

✗ DO NOT

- let the casualty rub the eye; this is a natural reaction to discomfort, but may make the condition worse.
- press on an injured eye.
- remove contact lenses unless rapid swelling is occurring, or you can't get prompt medical help.
- remove a foreign body that is resting on the cornea (the clear surface of the eye through which we see), or that appears to be embedded in any part of the eye.
- use dry cotton wool, cotton swabs or sharp instruments (such as tweezers) near the eye.
- risk contamination of a burn by breathing or coughing on it.

PREVENTION

- Wear protective goggles or safety spectacles when working with power tools or striking tools (such as hammers), to prevent objects flying into your eye.
- Only use garden sprays on a calm day, and wear protective goggles when spraying.
- When cutting trees or bushes, wear protective goggles as the sap of some plants can produce severe discomfort if it lands in your eyes.
- When working with toxic chemicals or any other substances that produce fumes, work in well-ventilated areas and wear protective goggles which seal the eye area.

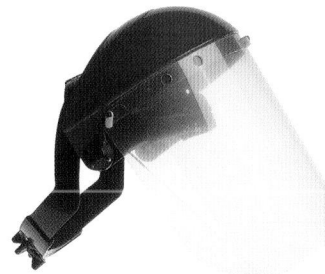

A full face mask will not only protect the eyes but the face as well.

Conjunctivitis (pink/red eye)

This an eye infection, as opposed to an environmentally based allergy or irritation. Conjunctivitis is characterized by severe burning and redness, with or without swelling of the eyelids and a yellow or greenish discharge. All eye infections are serious and should be seen by a doctor as soon as possible. In the interim, wash the eye with cool water and cover the closed eye with a cool cloth to help relieve the discomfort.

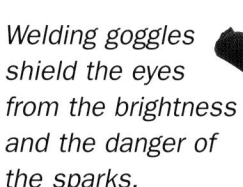

Welding goggles shield the eyes from the brightness and the danger of the sparks.

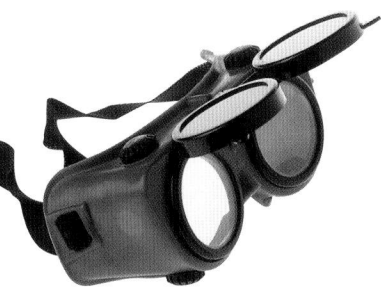

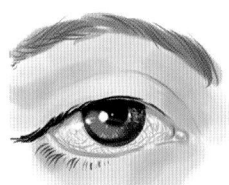

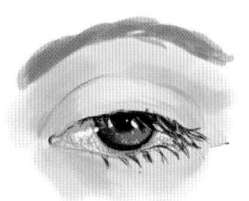

Viral conjunctivitis is also commonly known as 'pink eye'.

Bacterial conjunctivitis *causes gummy, sticky eyelashes.*

SEEK MEDICAL HELP IF:

- the eyeball appears scratched or has been penetrated by an object.
- a chemical has splashed into the eye.
- there is persistent pain and/or nausea.
- there are any vision problems.

Chest injuries

Chest injuries generally fall into two categories: penetrating or open wounds (where the skin is broken), and closed wounds (internal injuries). Treat them both as serious if the casualty is experiencing severe discomfort and/or shortness of breath

CAUSES

Closed chest injuries can occur when a motorist's chest hits the steering wheel as a result of an accident, for instance, or when a large heavy object, such as pipe or length of timber, slams into the casualty's chest. Such an accident can cause serious damage to the ribs, breast bone, heart or lungs.

Penetrating injuries include gunshots, stab wounds or penetration by other sharp objects.

SYMPTOMS

Closed chest injuries
- Pain
- Difficulty in breathing
- Shock due to loss of blood/oxygen
- Deformity or abnormal chest movement during breathing
- Bruising

Penetrating chest injuries
In addition to the above, these symptoms may also be present:
- A sucking sound as the casualty inhales
- Bubbling as the casualty exhales
- Bubbles in the blood around the wound

TAKE NOTE

- If an injury results in ribs being broken in more than one place, so that rib segments are able to move independently to some degree, the injured part of the chest wall tends to move abnormally (in when the casualty inhales, and out when they exhale). This is called a paradoxical chest movement and it makes breathing very difficult and painful.
- In extreme cases, an injury may cause one or both lungs to collapse; this condition, called pneumothorax, is life-threatening and must be treated as an emergency. This can happen with minimal trauma, and can occur spontaneously, in people with an inborn weakness or defect in their lungs (spontaneous pneumothorax).

TREATMENT

Call for an ambulance. Chest injuries are medical emergencies and must be assessed by a doctor.
- **Close off the wound to stop the flow of air through it**. If you do not have an airtight sterile dressing available, improvise with whatever is at hand, such as a clean plastic bag, or sandwich wrap for instance. Make a patch to cover the wound and tape it down on three sides only (*see* picture on p67). This will close when the casualty

inhales, admitting more air to the chest, and open when he or she exhales.

- Do not move the casualty if you suspect a head or spinal injury.
- If you have no reason to suspect a head or spinal injury, move the casualty into a semi-reclining position by propping them up. Lean them slightly towards the injured side so that the uninjured side is higher.
- If an embedded object (such as a piece of glass) caused the injury, do not remove it as you could do more damage. If feasible, support the object with a **ring bandage** (*see* p86).
- If a large object has caused a crushing chest injury, keep the casualty immobile while you wait for medical assistance.
- Loosen tight clothing, including belts or waist-bands.

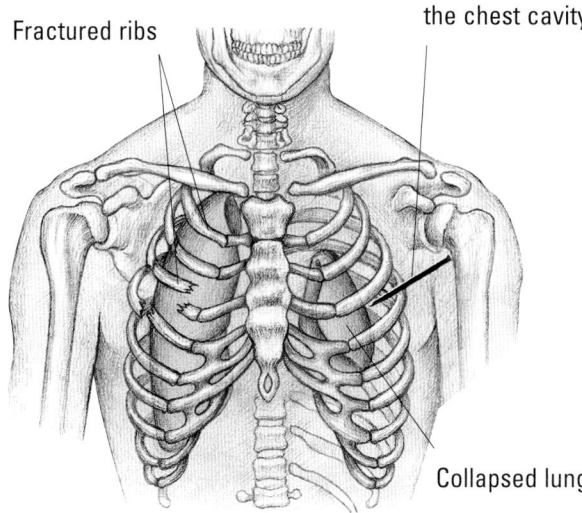

This illustration depicts two causes of chest injuries: on the right is a penetrating injury with a collapsed lung, while the left side depicts fractured ribs.

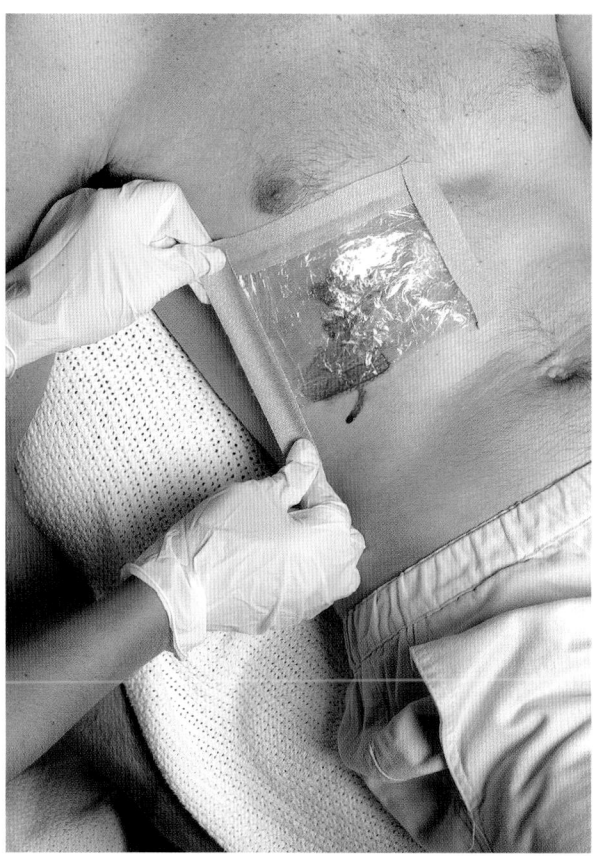

For an open chest injury, such as this puncture wound caused by an unfortunate fall, tape down the dressing on three sides. Leave one side open.

✗ DO NOT (also for p38)

- apply a tourniquet to control bleeding.
- lift the pad to see if bleeding has stopped, or replace a blood-soaked dressing. Just place a new one on top of it.
- probe an injury or try to remove a foreign object such as a knife.
- try to clean a large wound. This can cause heavier bleeding.
- try to clean an injury after you get the bleeding under control.

Fractures

A fracture is an injury to bone. A break results from the application of a force or stress that causes the bone to split or break. Stress fractures, usually small breaks, result when bone is subjected to repeated stress. A compound, or open, fracture occurs when the end of a broken bone breaks the skin and protrudes, or when the fracture results from a penetrating crush injury. Compound fractures must be treated immediately to prevent infection. As we age, our bones become brittle, which is why elderly people are more prone to fractures than younger people.

SYMPTOMS

- Limitation or unwillingness to move a limb
- Numbness and tingling
- Intense pain
- Bruising
- Swelling
- Inability to bear weight on a leg or use an arm
- Visibly out-of-place or misshapen limb or joint
- Bleeding or laceration (open fracture)

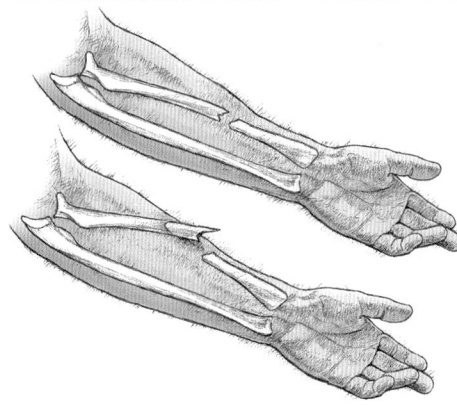

In a closed fracture (top), the bone does not penetrate the skin, as it does with an open, or compound, fracture (bottom).

CAUSES

- Direct blow to the bone.
- Falls, either from a height or on a slippery surface.
- Motor vehicle accidents.
- Excessive pressure.
- Stress fracture, from repetitive sports activity, for example.

TREATMENT

- In the case of a serious accident with the likelihood of broken bones, first **check the casualty's vital signs**. If it is necessary, begin **resuscitation** (*see* pp22–37), and control **bleeding** (*see* p38). Check for other life-threatening injuries, then keep the casualty still, provide reassurance, and call for medical help.
- **Keep the casualty warm**. Raise the feet about 30cm (12in), but do not move the casualty at all if a head, neck, or back injury is suspected.
- **In the case of an open, or compound fracture** try to gently rinse away any pieces of grass, bits of dirt and suchlike, but do not probe the wound, breathe on it or subject it to a vigorous scrubbing or flushing to remove the debris.
- **Cover open wounds with clean dressings** before immobilizing the injury (use a proprietary splint or improvise one from a rolled-up newspaper or piece of wood). Immobilize the area both above and below the injured bone, leaving it in the position in which it ended up.

SPLINTING FRACTURES BELOW THE ELBOW

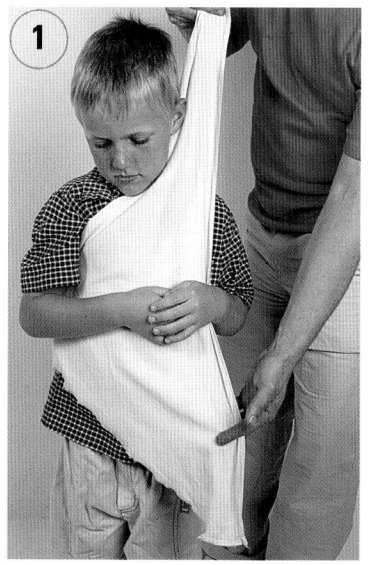 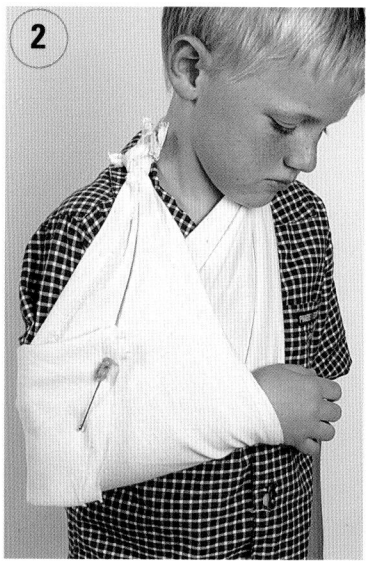

1. *Prepare a triangular bandage while the child supports the injured arm. Always apply the sling or bandage to the arm in whichever position you find it. Then tie the ends securely so that the knot does not rub against and irritate the back of the neck.*

2. *Do not bend the elbow beyond 90 degrees as bone fragments can press on the nerves and vessels that run just in front of the elbow and may interfere with blood flow. For the same reason you should never apply any sling or dressing that encircles the arm tightly at any point.*

- **Check that circulation is still healthy below the fracture**. For instance, in the case of a broken arm, press your fingertip on the casualty's finger for five seconds. The area should turn pale and then regain its normal colour within three seconds. If it does not, or there is numbness, lack of a pulse and pale or blue skin, the circulation is inadequate. Splint the fracture in the position in which you find it and get the casualty to a hospital as soon as possible.
- If an open fracture is bleeding, place a clean, dry cloth over the wound. **If the bleeding continues, apply direct pressure** to the site of bleeding, taking care not to apply any pressure to the protruding end of the bone.
- **Summon medical assistance** as soon as possible. In the case of a broken ankle or arm, get the casualty to an emergency room.

PREVENTION

- Wear the recommended protective gear while engaged in an active sport or pastime.
- Create a safe environment for young children and supervise them properly no matter how safe the situation appears to be. Help children learn how to look out for themselves and teach them basic safety techniques.
- Avoid falls by taking care when walking on wet, slippery or icy surfaces, and observing posted warnings.
- Use handrails when going up and down stairs and getting on and off escalators.
- Ensure that ladders are secure when doing household maintenance or gardening.
- Some people are reluctant to use a cane or walking aid, but it is far better to suffer some loss of dignity than deal with the aftermath of a broken limb or hip.

EASY SLING FOR FRACTURES ABOVE THE ELBOW

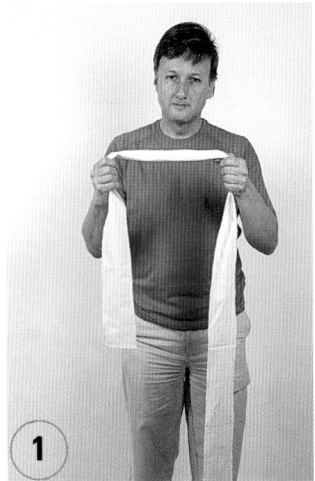

1 Grab a 1m (3ft) length of flannel or linen. Hold it away from the centre in such a way that you have one long end and one shorter end.

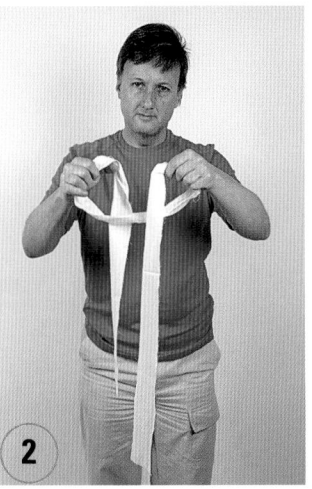

2 Fold two loops as shown; the longer one looping behind and the shorter one in front of the central piece.

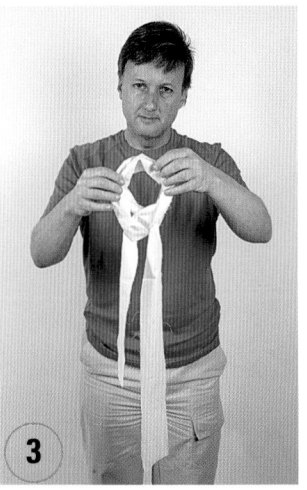

3 Superimpose the two loops (fold them together) to form a clove hitch.

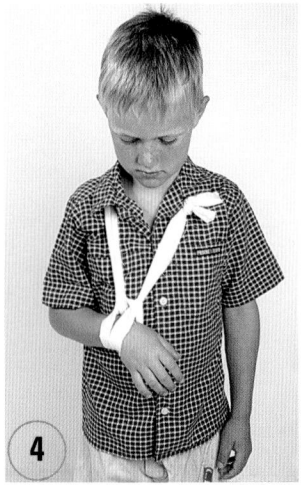

4 Place the double loops around the wrist of the injured arm and tie the ends together.

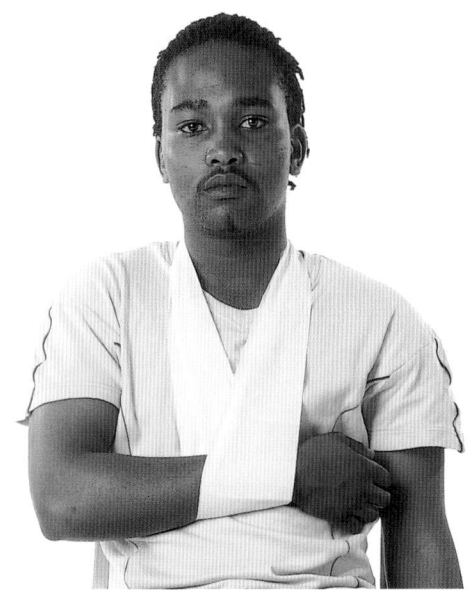

An alternative method of strapping an upper limb. Use a triangular bandage and a strip of flannel or linen to immobilize an arm or shoulder injury until the casualty can be taken to an emergency room.

X DO NOT

- move the casualty if a head, spine or back injury is suspected. In the case of a fractured hip, pelvis or upper leg, move the casualty only if absolutely necessary (for example out of harm's way following a road accident). Do so by pulling the casualty by their clothing, not by any limbs, which could also be injured.
- move the casualty unless the injury is completely immobilized. Never try to reposition a suspected cervical spine injury.
- try to straighten a misshapen bone or joint, or change its position.
- test a misshapen bone or joint for loss of function.
- give the casualty anything by mouth.
- apply a tourniquet to the extremity to stop the bleeding. Apply direct pressure.

SPLINTING FRACTURES BELOW THE KNEE

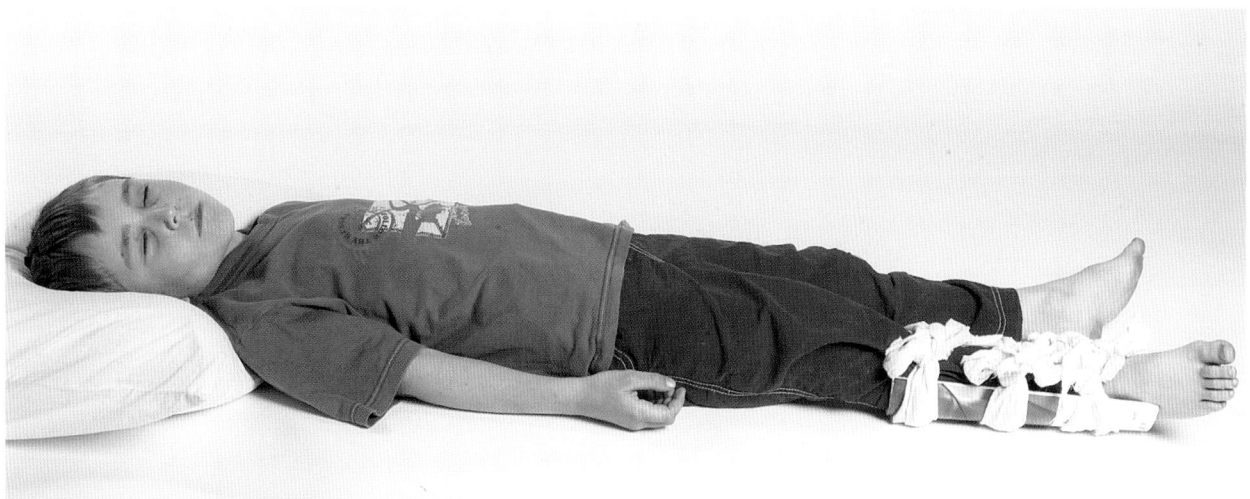

If you have called the ambulance, simply support the calf with a pillow, a rolled-up towel or blanket. If you have to transport the child yourself, you can splint the lower leg with a rolled magazine, newspaper or any sturdy object which extends a few inches above the knee and below the ankle. Foot injuries do not need splinting, particularly if the child is small enough for you to carry.

Pain relief – Pain at the fracture site is mostly due to the broken bone ends rubbing against each other. This can be minimized by splinting the limb and letting the child move as little as possible.

SPLINTING FRACTURES ABOVE THE KNEE

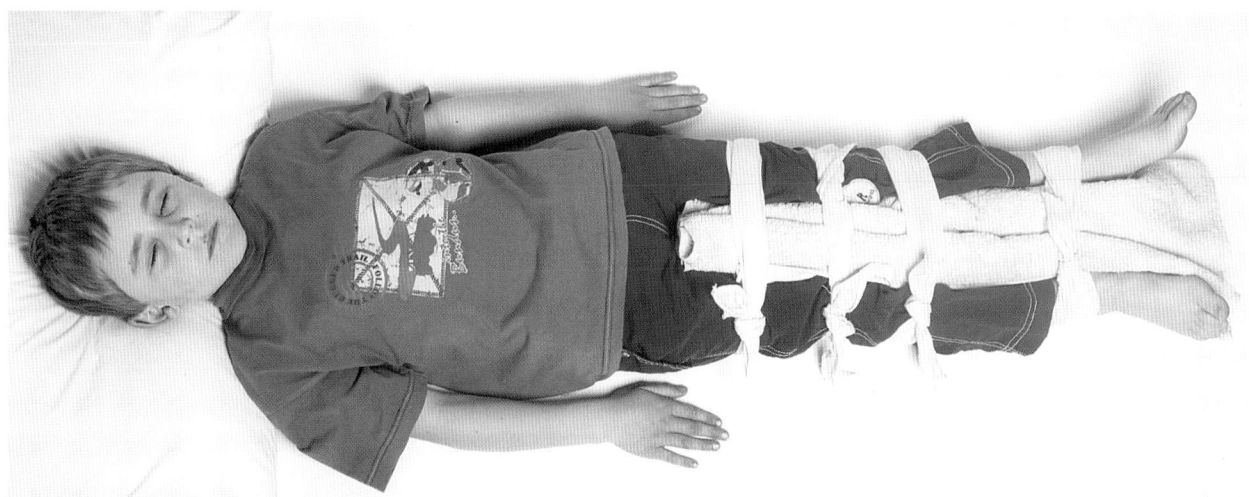

Splint the injured leg to the opposite limb using four 1m (3ft) lengths of linen, flannel or adhesive plaster. Do not move the casualty; wait for the ambulance to arrive and allow the ambulance staff to move him.

Sprains and strains (muscle, tendon and ligament injuries)

The terms 'strain' and 'sprain' refer to injuries caused by overstretching or tearing a muscle, tendon or ligament. These are uncommon before adolescence because the developing bones of children are more susceptible to injury than the neighbouring soft tissues. Consequently, strains and sprains should only be diagnosed in children once fractures or joint injuries have been excluded beyond doubt by X-ray examination. The fully developed bone of adults is reinforced with calcium, so that injury to the muscles, tendons and ligaments occur more frequently, particularly in an active person who frequently indulges in a variety of sports, exercise or exertion. (*See also* **fractures**, p68).

SYMPTOMS

- Sudden severe pain or cramp at the site of injury
- Aggravation of pain by any degree of movement at the site of injury
- Swelling directly over the injury. This is greatest with torn muscle which has a rich blood supply, however bruising only becomes visible in the days after injury

CAUSES

Even at rest, low-level nerve impulses ensure that muscles and their tendons remain semi-taut and in a state of readiness, prepared to act in response to the body's needs.

Any sudden, violent movement for which the muscles or tendons are unprepared, can cause them to tear, causing bleeding, pain and loss of function. This happens most frequently during vigorous exercise or contact sport, or if a fall onto an outstretched arm or leg results in sudden, involuntary stretching or bending of the limb.

Ligaments are short, fibrous bands which run between neighbouring bones, to reinforce joint capsules. They may be stretched and damaged by forcibly moving a joint beyond its normal range, or as part of a deeper joint injury caused by a fall, sports injury or motor vehicle collision.

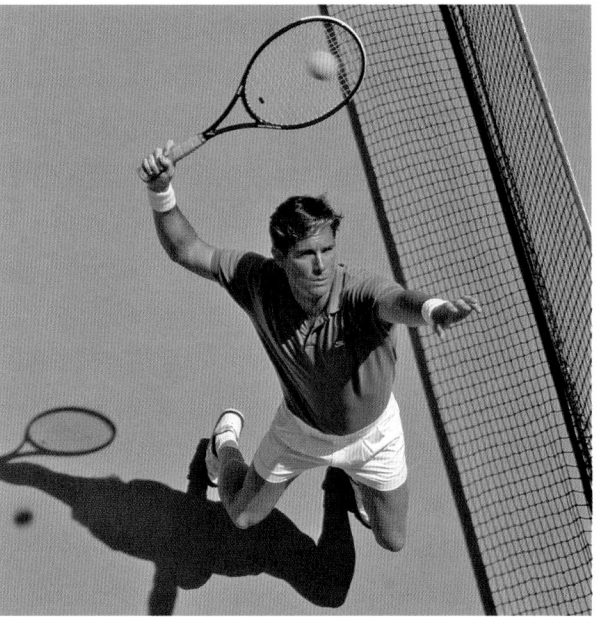

Vigorous exercise can cause a tendon or ligament to stretch or tear.

HOW TO MAKE A COLD COMPRESS

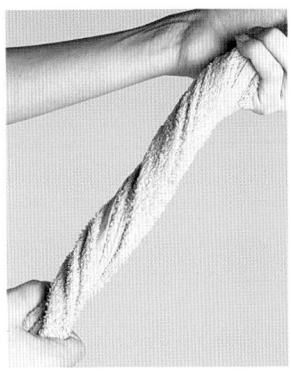 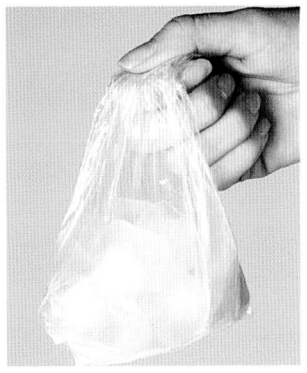

1. *Wring out a wet hand towel.*

2. *Fill a bag with ice.*

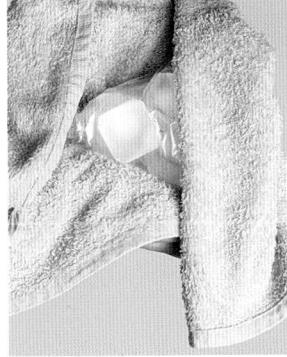 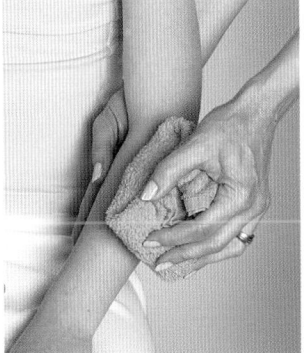

3. *Wrap the ice in the damp towel.*

4. *Apply the compress to the affected area.*

TREATMENT

- Let casualty sit or lie down.
- Follow the **RICE** principle: rest the affected limb; apply a cold compress and keep it in place for 10 minutes. Repeat if necessary. Elevate the injured limb, supporting it in the most comfortable position by using a pillow or rolled-up item of clothing.
- **Use splints** to keep movement of the injured limb to a minimum (*see* **fractures** p68).
- If pain persists despite splinting, **a painkiller may be administered** orally (500mg for older children, 1000mg for adults).
- **Seek medical attention** to confirm the diagnosis and provide definitive treatment. Sprains and fractures may occur together, so suspected injuries should be X-rayed.

- Do not delay application of a **cold compress** for the sake of rubbing on ointments or lotions. With a sprain, nothing is quicker or more efficient than ice to keep swelling and bleeding to a minimum.
- Do not treat sprains and strains with just an elasticated bandage around the injured area, as this will do little to limit movement. Torn ligaments and tendons may require rigid immobilization in a plaster cast or even surgical repair. A doctor must take the decision regarding the correct management of the injury.

PREVENTION

- Sports participants should ensure that they are sufficiently fit for their sport. Being a good runner doesn't mean you won't suffer an arm or shoulder injury if you play a vigorous game of tennis.
- Always warm up properly before beginning any exercise or sport, and take care not to get chilled during exercise.
- If you sustain a sprain or strain during sport or exercise, allow time for complete healing to take place before you become active again. Continued aggravation may turn a minor injury into a major one, while repeat injuries can result in delayed or incomplete healing, or even permanent weakness of the tendon or ligament. Once the injury has healed, start slowly and build up gradually before returning to your previous level of activity.
- When working up a ladder, or at any height above ground level, ensure that you are securely positioned at all times to prevent yourself from falling (*see* p145).

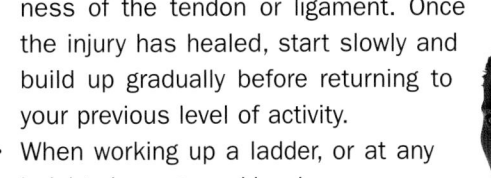 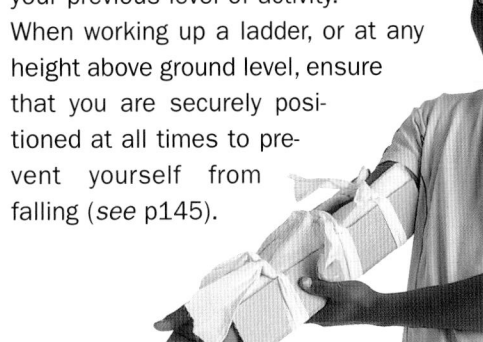

This forearm splint has been improvised from cardboard and soft dressing materials.

Neck, back and spinal cord injuries

The spine, or vertebral column, has two important functions: it is the central 'strut' of the skeleton around which all movement occurs, and it encases and protects the spinal cord along which nerve impulses are conducted to and from the brain to all parts of the body. It is this second function which concerns us most in the event of injury. Any fracture or displacement of one or more vertebrae can compress, tear or sever the spinal cord, causing partial or total paralysis of the body below the level of injury. When providing first aid, always consider the possibility of spinal injury and take the necessary precautions to avoid aggravating any injury which may already be present.

SYMPTOMS

- Unconscious casualty: always assume a spinal injury at first, particularly if there is also evidence of a head injury.
- Conscious casualty: may complain of pain at the site of a back injury; in the case of neck injury they may hold their neck rigidly to one side.
- Damage to the spinal cord may cause weakness of all or some muscles below the level of the injury, giving a sense of numbness (pins and needles).
- Damage to the spinal cord in the neck region may cause paralysis of the chest muscles and diaphragm, making it difficult for the casualty to breathe normally.
- Blood vessels below the level of spinal cord injury lose their normal tone, so that blood pressure drops. This is known as 'spinal shock', and should be suspected in any casualty who appears to be paralysed.
- Severe spinal cord injury may affect bladder functioning.

CAUSES

Most spinal injuries in young people result from high-velocity impact, such as car accidents, contact sports and falls from a height. However, the spine may also be injured in accidents which occur around the home, such as falling off a ladder or diving into a shallow swimming pool. Elderly people can sustain spinal injuries from relatively minor trauma such as a fall, purely because their vertebrae and the discs between them are more brittle and less able to absorb the shock of even a minor impact.

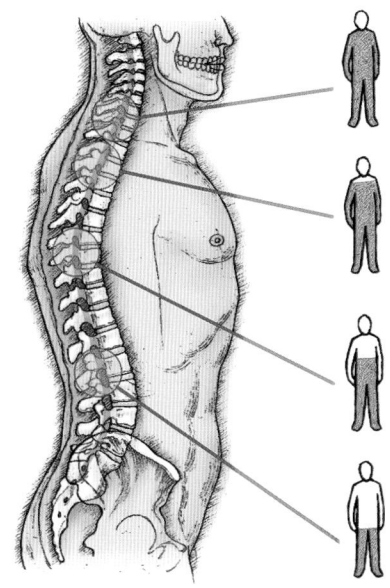

Depending on the site of an injury to the spinal cord, different parts of the body are affected.

TREATMENT

- **If you suspect a spinal injury**, call for an ambulance or the emergency services immediately.

- **If the casualty is unconscious**, assess the **ABC** (*see* pp22–3) and then commence **resuscitation** (*see* pp22–37) if necessary.

- If providing resuscitation, steady the neck with the same hand which pinches the nostrils closed. **Always maintain the neck in whichever position you find it**.

- If you have a second person to assist with first aid, they should stabilize the neck with two hands while you proceed with resuscitation.

- **A casualty who is conscious and breathing, but complains of neck or back pain**, should remain on his back until the emergency services arrive. Support the neck using a solid, heavy object, such as a brick placed on either side of the head. If something solid is not available, continue to support the head and neck gently but firmly with your hands.

⚠ CAUTION

- Don't give the casualty anything to eat or drink as they are likely to vomit it up.
- Don't try to straighten the spine if you find the casualty lying at an angle; you may cause more damage.
- Be extremely cautious about raising the legs to treat shock, particularly if there is any sign that the pelvis or lower back may be injured. Raising the legs may aggravate the injury and also cause severe pain.

PREVENTION

- Any child under eight years old should be supervised by an adult when near any body of water.
- Do not permit children to dive into shallow pools, or any water where the depth, or the presence of submerged objects, is unknown.
- During home DIY activities, ensure that your ladders are in a good state of repair, securely positioned on level surfaces, and long enough for the job in hand to be performed safely.
- Elderly people, particularly those with failing vision or who may be unsteady on their feet, should be escorted, or use walking aids when negotiating unfamiliar territory, especially steps or staircases.
- In contact sports such as rugby football, gridiron and ice hockey, neck injuries are less likely if the teams are appropriately matched, and if referees strictly apply the rules of the game.

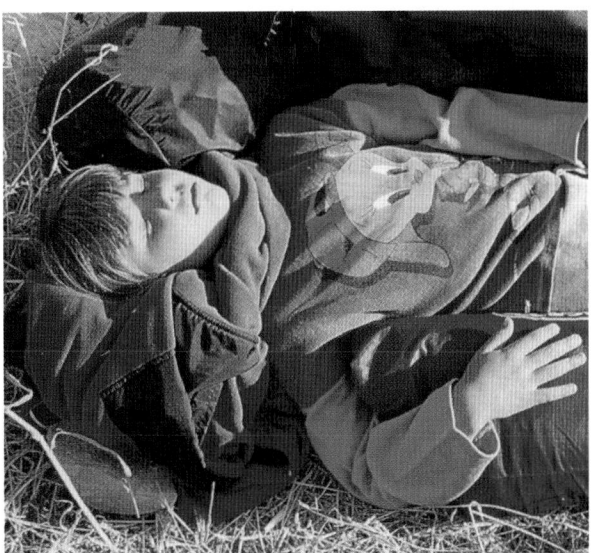

If the neck is stiffly held in one position, leave it as it is. Carefully support the neck by placing a heavy object on either side until the patient is fully awake. Do not force him or her to straighten a stiff neck, as this may well aggravate an underlying injury.

HOME CARE

The ability to provide effective first aid in the home may save you a visit to a hospital or doctor's rooms when minor injuries or illnesses occur. In this section, we describe a range of basic skills and techniques which, together with a well-stocked first aid kit (*see* pp14–5), will enable you to treat a range of minor conditions with confidence. You will also learn which symptoms are serious enough to require medical assistance.

In any family group, it is the very young and the elderly who are most vulnerable to injury, and who create the greatest anxiety when they are unwell. This section covers a range of minor childhood problems, but the scope of our recommendations is limited by the fact that no two children react identically to the same illness. Symptoms and signs may vary, therefore, if doubt exists regarding a diagnosis or suitability of home care, we urge the first-aid provider to seek medical advice without delay.

Managing injuries in small children requires patience and steady nerves. Some are so distressed that any attempt at first aid risks becoming a battle of wills. In such cases, prudence is certainly the better part of valour, and medical assistance should be sought.

Elderly family members are prone to injury due to failing eyesight, brittle bones and unsteady gait, or may require ongoing home nursing. Rather than attempt to cover the full range of medical conditions which may trouble the elderly, we offer practical suggestions on day-to-day home nursing and frail care in the final chapter of this section.

IN THIS SECTION

Chest pains

Not all chest pain signifies a heart attack, but a systematic first aid approach will allow you to determine whether a particular type of chest pain signals a life-threatening episode, and how best to react. Chest pain is not an uncommon occurrence, but it creates justifiably more cause for concern in adults – particularly those with a family history of heart disease and those known to be exposed to certain risk factors (i.e. high blood pressure, or smoking). Chest pain that occurs without warning may be a symptom of a variety of conditions. The significance of the pain depends not only on its severity, but on the presence or absence of associated symptoms (see panel below).

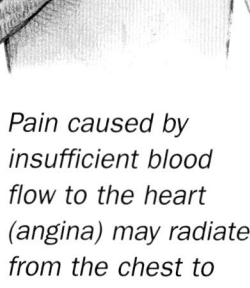

Pain caused by insufficient blood flow to the heart (angina) may radiate from the chest to the neck and arms.

SYMPTOMS

In all cases of chest pain it is advisable to seek medical help immediately.

- Severe, prolonged pain which does not go away with rest, or causes the casualty to go into **shock** (*see* p40), strongly indicates the likelihood of a heart attack.
- Sharp, sudden pain in the upper chest or back, accompanied by signs of shock, may be due to blood leaking from a diseased aorta.
- A sense of pressure or heaviness over the breastbone that is triggered by either physical exertion or emotional stress is likely to be angina.

- A stabbing pain felt in any part of the chest wall, and aggravated by deep breathing or coughing, may be due to an inflammation in the chest cavity, especially if the person also has a mild fever.
- Burning pain in the lower chest, especially after meals, may signify acid reflux associated with hiatus hernia. It is often relieved by antacids.
- Sharp, stabbing pains in the lower chest after persistent or violent bouts of vomiting may indicate a tear in the oesophageal lining, particularly if streaks of fresh red blood appear in the vomit.

- Sudden, deep discomfort while eating solid food, sometimes accompanied by difficulty breathing and excess salivation, could be due to abnormal or delayed peristalsis (the normal movement of the oesophagus) or by food becoming impacted at any point in the mid- or lower oesophagus.
- If chest pain is caused by an injury to the chest wall (by blunt or penetrating trauma), emergency first aid should follow the recommendations for **chest injuries** on p66.

CAUSES

- **Cardiovascular** Chest pain may signify heart strain (angina), from early or advanced coronary artery disease, heart attack, infection or inflammation of the heart muscle (myocarditis) or the thin sac surrounding the heart (pericarditis), or leakage of blood from the aorta.
- **Respiratory system** Although pain is seldom a major feature of lung or airway infection, severe chest pains experienced during breathing may be caused by an infection spreading to the pleura (the thin membrane covering each lung and lining the chest cavity).
- **Digestive system** Chest pain may be caused by stomach acid leaking into the lower oesophagus (gullet), a frequent symptom in people with hiatus hernia. Simply eating too fast may cause solid food to impact on the mid- or lower oesophagus, with temporary pain or discomfort. Repeated vomiting for any reason can tear the delicate lining of the oesophagus.
- **The chest wall** The muscles of the chest wall may be torn or sprained by physical exertion, causing either immediate discomfort, or chest pain which only becomes obvious after a few hours. Certain viruses, which cause flu-like illnesses, may cause an inflammation of the intercostal muscles (between the ribs), resulting in sharp, localized pain on breathing, two to five days after other symptoms of the illness have disappeared.

TREATMENT

Although it helps to establish the likely cause of chest pain if possible, the focus of first aid is to recognize what – mainly cardiovascular – causes are life-threatening, then to call for assistance, and to provide supportive treatment while you wait for help.

If you suspect that the casualty has had a heart attack – and until an ambulance or your doctor arrives – you can:

- Give them 1 soluble disprin to dissolve slowly under the tongue.

 DO NOT

- give the casualty anything by mouth, other than prescribed heart medication.
- leave the casualty alone, except to call an ambulance.
- wait to see if the symptoms disappear without intervention.

 SEEK MEDICAL HELP IMMEDIATELY:

- If the casualty loses consciousness or stops breathing. Commence resuscitation (see pp22–37) and continue until help arrives.
- If the casualty shows any signs of shock (see p40) or has trouble breathing. Cover him with a blanket to reduce heat loss and wait for help to arrive. Calmly comfort and reassure an anxious person if necessary.
- If the casualty is known to suffer from heart disease or has had a previous heart attack.
- If pain which appears after effort, and which is possibly cardiac in origin, does not improve immediately with rest.
- If blood is coughed or vomited up after the onset of pain.
- If the casualty suffers from a heart condition and has medication handy, provide assistance to take it (usually a tablet that is placed under the tongue). The pain should subside within three minutes of taking the medication and resting; then summon medical assistance immediately.

PREVENTING HEART DISEASE

You can reduce the risk of heart disease by:

- Avoiding smoking.
- Keeping your weight within the recommended range for your height.
- Maintaining a balanced, low-fat diet.
- Moderating your alcohol intake.
- Engaging in physical activity three times a week for 20 minutes.
- Having annual check-ups and blood cholesterol measurements from age 40 onwards.
- Having annual check-ups from age 30 if heart disease is prevalent in your family.

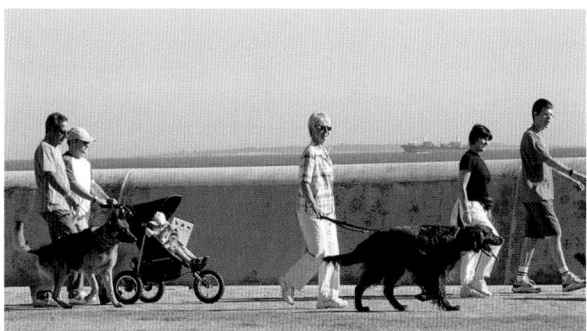

COMMON HEART CONDITIONS

- **Angina,** an inadequate supply of blood to the heart muscle, causes pain that radiates to the neck, shoulder, or arms, accompanied by sudden fatigue, shortness of breath or palpitations. Angina usually improves with rest, or by placing isordil nitrate tablets under the tongue.
- **Hiatus hernia** is a protrusion of the stomach into the chest cavity. This common condition can be successfully treated with weight loss, medication or 'key-hole' surgery. See your doctor if persistent symptoms occur after meals, or interfere with routine eating habits.
- **Hypertension,** persistent high blood pressure, puts strain on the arteries and heart, resulting in damage that occurs over time. Termed the 'silent killer', it has no symptoms.

Regular exercise such as walking or jogging will tone your body and reduce the likelihood of heart disease.

Stroke

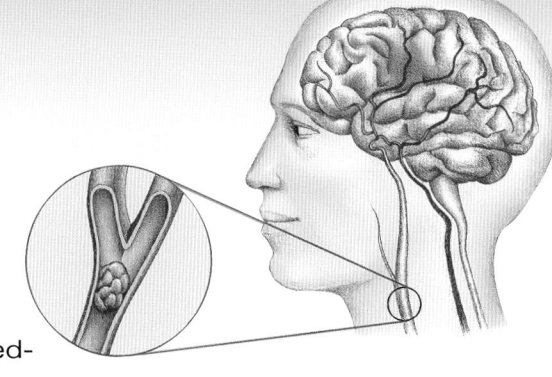

Strokes are a major cause of death in many developed countries, and result in significant disability among survivors. Also known as cerebrovascular accidents (CVAs), strokes can be caused by a haemorrhage (bleeding) from an artery in the brain (a process called cerebral thrombosis), or when atherosclerosis plaques (fatty deposits and blood clots) migrate from another part of the body and lodge in the carotid artery that supplies blood to the brain (*see* illustration). A stroke is therefore an interruption of the blood supply to any part of the brain. If the interruption is longer than a few seconds, brain cells can die resulting in permanent damage.

The symptoms depend on the severity of the stroke and the part of the brain that is damaged. Some may even be unaware that they have suffered a minor stroke. In others, both symptoms and long term effects are severe. Generally, the symptoms develop suddenly:

- Loss of movement (paralysis) or co-ordination of any body area, including the face
- Numbness, weakness, loss of sensation or tingling in the limbs, particularly on one side of the body
- Dizziness or vertigo (a sensation of movement), possibly leading to a fall
- Impaired vision, drooping or uncontrolled eye movements
- Drooling or swallowing difficulties
- Loss of ability to identify certain stimuli
- Slurred speech or the inability to speak, or understand speech
- Changes in levels of consciousness (e.g. sleepy or lethargic, comatose or faint)
- Loss of memory

CAUSES

Strokes often result from atherosclerosis. Blood platelets and fatty deposits collect on the artery walls and, over time, obstruct the flow more and more. If the deposit stays where it formed and blocks the artery, it is known as a thrombus. If it breaks free and blocks a vessel elsewhere, it is called an embolus.

Heart disorders such as an irregular heart rate, may cause a stroke, depriving the brain of blood and oxygen. Ailments such as diabetes and hypertension can also contribute to the onset of a stroke.

Although men are generally more at risk, certain factors increase a woman's risk over the age of 35.

Most notably, these include a combination of smoking and taking certain birth control pills, or other medication that promotes clot formation.

TREATMENT

If the casualty does not lose consciousness, or the symptoms are transient:

- Reassure the casualty.
- Avoid any physical exertion; keep the casualty sedated and monitor the heart beat.
- Do not administer any medication, whether prescribed or otherwise.
- Observe the casualty until all of the symptoms are totally resolved.
- Seek medical advice without delay.

If the casualty is unconscious, has difficulty breathing or is unable to move:

- Call for medical help immediately.
- Check their airway (remove loose dentures, food or any other obstruction in the mouth).
- If the casualty is not breathing, commence **resuscitation** (*see* pp22–37) and continue until help arrives.
- Ensure that all known information regarding regular medications is conveyed to the hospital via the emergency staff.
- Do not give the casualty any food or drink, as the swallowing mechanism may be paralysed, risking aspiration into the lungs.

PREVENTION

Lead a healthy lifestyle and modify your habits to reduce high alcohol consumption, excessive smoking and lack of exercise. Take prescribed medication for conditions such as high blood pressure, diabetes or high cholesterol. If you are over the age of 40 ensure that you have regular medical assessments annually. Begin this earlier if you have a known family history of conditions such as high blood pressure, high cholesterol, heart attacks or strokes. (*See also* Preventing Heart Disease p80.)

Preventing infection

Once the protective skin barrier that surrounds the human body is disturbed or broken, bacteria can invade and there is a risk of infection. In order to prevent infections you must ensure that wounds are cleaned thoroughly and all germs and dirt removed using an antiseptic dilute (chlorhexidin or povidone-iodine). Do your best to keep a fresh wound free of moisture for at least 48 hours. It is not necessary to change the dressings every day unless they become soiled; in any event, doing so may do more harm than good because it can disturb the scar and thus cause delayed healing. Dressings that remain clean and intact can be removed after seven days, and need only be replaced if the wound still appears raw. Wet, bloody or tattered dressings should be replaced swiftly to prevent infection.

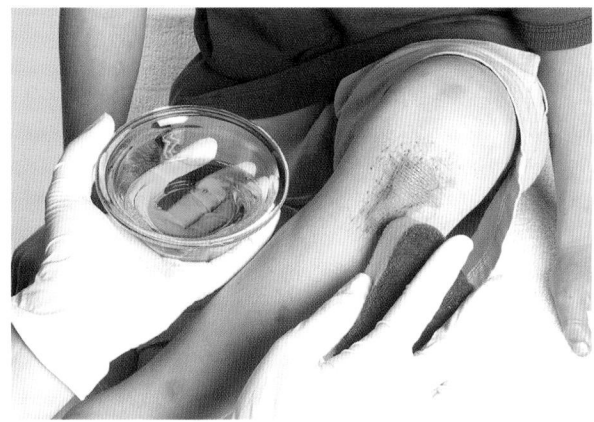

To reduce the risk of infection, wash all wounds thoroughly with a mild antiseptic solution.

TIP

Always wash your hands thoroughly before you begin any first aid. To guard against the risk of infection, use surgical gloves when blood or bodily fluids are involved.

TREATMENT

- **Stop the bleeding:** Many small wounds stop bleeding on their own. More vigorous bleeding can be controlled with direct pressure for a few minutes, using a clean dressing or cloth. Wash all open wounds with water and a dilute antiseptic solution. Even if the wound appears clean to your naked eye, you can safely assume that dirt is present and must be washed out. Injured hands, feet and limbs can be washed under cold water for two minutes. Wounds on other parts of the body can be washed with a clean cloth dipped in antiseptic solution.
- **Cleaning:** Carefully remove all dirt and foreign matter still visible in the wound after washing. Wipe the wound gently but firmly with a soft clean kitchen sponge dipped in dilute antiseptic solution. Then use a clean pair of tweezers or forceps to pick out any ingrained dirt which remains. If a flap of skin has been lifted over the cut, be sure to wash and clean well underneath it. Wounds with deeply ingrained soil or dirt that is difficult to remove may require cleaning under a local anaesthetic. In such cases, cover the wound with a clean dressing or cloth and go to see your nearest hospital or emergency room.

DRESSING WOUNDS

Dressings should protect a fresh wound from re-injury and infection. Tiny cuts and abrasions which are not actively bleeding may be left open, lightly dabbed with antiseptic ointment or cream (such as Dettol, Savlon or Betadine) or simply covered with an adhesive plaster.

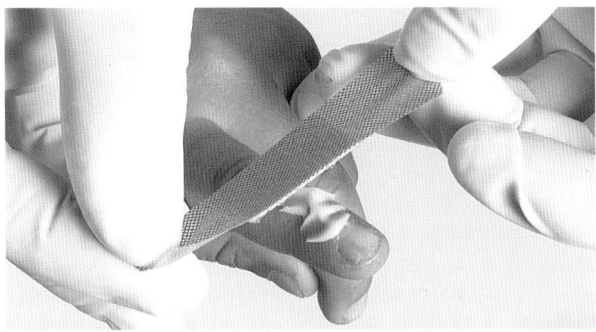

The mildest injury requires only a dab of antiseptic ointment and an adhesive plaster.

All dressings consist of two components: a non-sticky pad or swab to cover the wound, and a secure bandage or adhesive plaster to keep the pad in place. Paraffin-impregnated gauze (Jelonet) is a versatile dressing for any raw or burnt area of skin. A single layer of paraffin gauze is sufficient to cover most wounds.

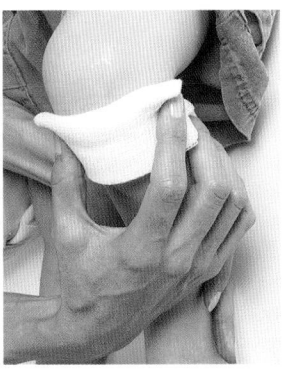

Place a swab over the wound then ...

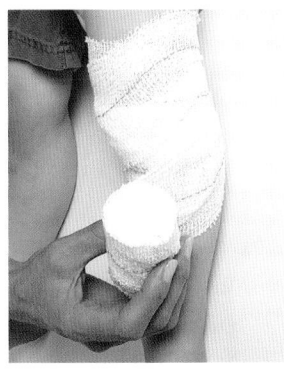

... bandage to keep the swab in place.

✗ DO NOT

- use cotton wool to dress raw wounds, as the fibres will become embedded in the scar, making removal very painful.
- apply powdery substances, foodstuffs or household cleaning agents to an open wound. Use only what is recommended, or nothing at all.

SEEK MEDICAL HELP IF:

- Wounds have not been washed and cleaned within six hours of injury.
- Wounds appear infected: surrounding skin is red and puffy; there is increasing pain; there is a yellowish discharge.
- It is a punture wound, particularly if an animal or human bite has broken the skin.
- The wound requires stitches.
- A penetrating wound has occurred below the wrist (risk of tendon or nerve injury).
- Lips or the eyes are wounded.
- There is bruising around the eye socket.
- A wound continues to bleed despite adequate pressure (*see below*).

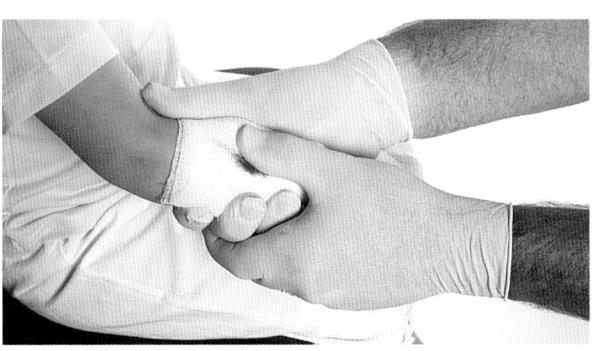

Cuts, grazes, bruises and lacerations

Cuts, grazes and bruises are everyday occurrences, particularly with children, but can easily be treated at home with the help of antiseptic cleaning agents, dressings and bandages. Most cuts heal quickly and completely, but a common complication is infection, which can delay healing and cause scarring. Therefore, the priority for first-aid treatment is to clean all wounds as quickly and thoroughly as possible, using basic principles of hygiene.

SYMPTOMS

- **Cuts, lacerations and puncture wounds:** These may be clean cuts or ragged injuries. With deeper cuts particularly, there is a risk of infection if the wound is not properly cleaned. Pain, swelling, or a yellowish discharge are all signs of infection.

- **Abrasions:** The scraped area of skin is painful and appears dark pink or red. Bleeding varies according to the depth of the abrasion. Dirt may be embedded in damaged skin, depending on what surface was scraped against.

- **Bruises:** A fresh bruise is very tender to touch, and may or may not cause swelling under the skin. As it heals, a bruise changes colour from reddish-purple to green to yellow over a period of five to seven days, disappearing within 10 days.

TREATMENT FOR CUTS AND GRAZES

- **Wash** with mild soap and warm water, or a solution of mild antiseptic liquid and water, to remove any obvious loose debris or dirt from a superficial injury (one that affects the surface of the skin only).

- **For grazes** (not for cuts), pat **dry and apply antiseptic ointment**, and **dress** with a plaster or sterile dressing

- **For cuts**, pat **dry**, and **dress** with a plaster or sterile dressing

- **Do not probe** a wound for embedded objects or debris. You may cause more damage. Rather leave it as is and get it treated immediately.

- If muscle, tissue or bone have been exposed, do not push them back into place. Simply **bandage or dress** the wound and get the casualty to an emergency room.

- If you suspect a deep wound may require stitches, **take the patient to a doctor** or hospital room as soon as possible.

- Consult your doctor if an infection is not cured or becomes worse.

CAUSES

- **Cuts and lacerations:** A cut is an injury in which the skin has been opened. Cuts have clean edges, lacerations are jagged wounds or tears.
- **Puncture wounds:** These can be from scissors, pins, or splinters, for instance, to those caused by large objects such as tools or kitchen utensils. Animal bites can result in deep puncture wounds.
- **Abrasions:** The superficial outer layers of the skin may be accidentally scraped as a result of a fall or a slide along any rough surface.
- **Bruises:** Usually caused by blunt force such as a fall, bumping into something, being hit by a moving object. The skin remains intact, but damage to blood vessels causes bleeding under the skin.

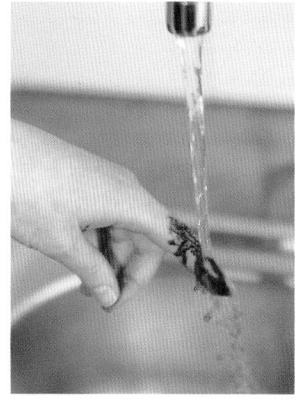

Wash a cut under a running tap to remove blood and dirt.

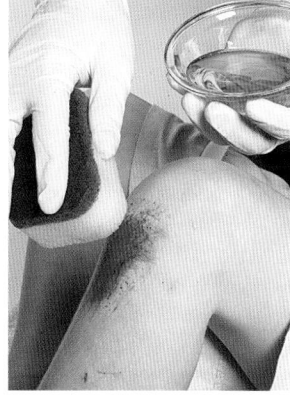

A graze can be cleaned with a sponge dipped in diluted antiseptic.

 DO NOT

- clean a large wound or try to clean it if bleeding has stopped. In the first instance you may make the bleeding worse, and in the latter, you may restart it.
- attempt first-aid remedies that may have to be undone before proper treatment can take place. If you suspect that a wound will require stitches, simply apply a clean, lint-free bandage or dressing to contain the bleeding and get the casualty to the doctor or emergency room.
- encircle a finger, arm or leg with any tight plaster or bandage which could interfere with the blood supply.

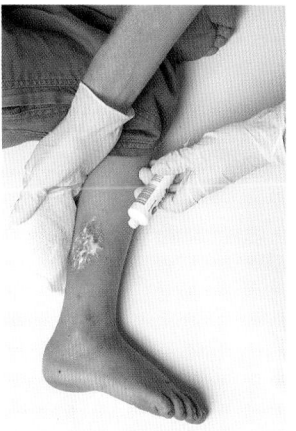

Only use antiseptic ointment on grazes before dressing.

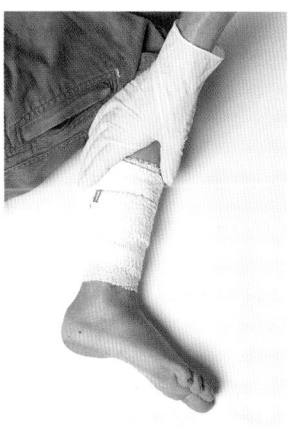

Dress a cut or graze with a plaster or a clean bandage.

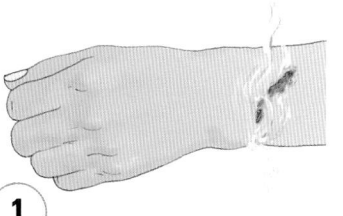

1 *Wash the wound*

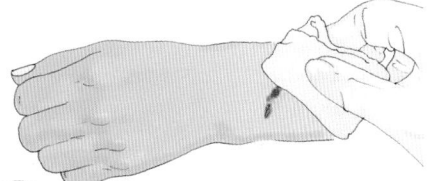

2 *Clean carefully and gently.*

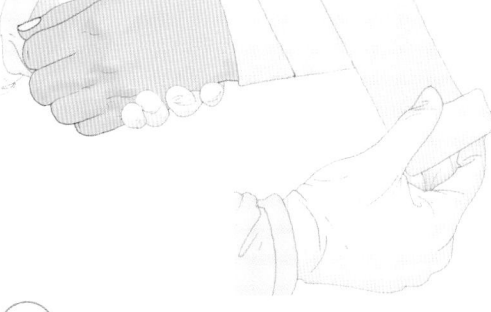

3 *Apply dressing.*

LACERATIONS

- Rinse, then wash the wound thoroughly with mild soap and water.
- Control **bleeding** (*see* p38).
- Cover the wound with a butterfly bandage.
- If the laceration looks serious, consult your doctor.

PUNCTURE WOUNDS

- Rinse and then clean the wound with mild soap and flowing water – to try to wash out any fragments of whatever caused the injury.
- Apply a clean bandage.
- Get medical assistance.

EMBEDDED OBJECTS

- Apart from splinters and objects of a similar size, do not remove an object that is embedded in the skin, particularly one that has penetrated deeply – doing so can cause more damage and initiate bleeding if the object has penetrated a major blood vessel.
- Make up a ring bandage, place it over the object without touching it, and bandage it into position to prevent it from moving laterally. Do not move the object or apply any downward pressure to it. You will need to carry out this manoeuvre extremely carefully as the object should be kept absolutely still with relation to whatever part of the body it has penetrated.
- Call for assistance or get the casualty to a hospital or doctor immediately.

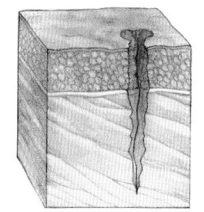 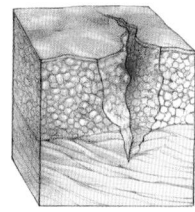

The entry of a puncture wound is neat, but the wound can go deep into the muscle.

Lacerations are usually fairly shallow but have wider openings and jagged edges.

TETANUS

Tetanus, sometimes known as lockjaw, is a life-threatening infection. The bacterial organism responsible is particularly widespread in manure and other animal waste. Once tetanus bacteria enter the body through an open wound, they target the spinal cord, releasing a toxin that causes severe spasms and difficulty in breathing. If left untreated, death can occur from heart or lung failure. Tetanus is extremely difficult to treat once symptoms appear as it does not respond to antibiotics. Children are routinely immunized by standard vaccination schedules.

APPLYING A RING BANDAGE

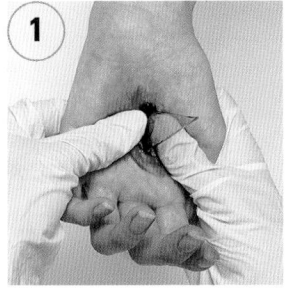 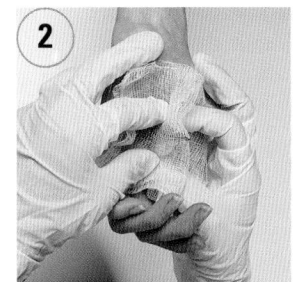 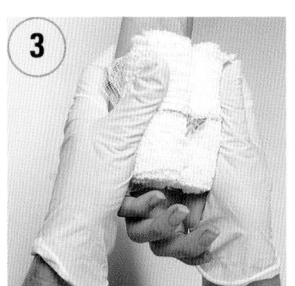 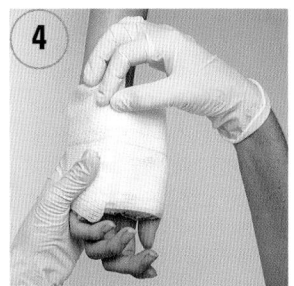

1. *Pinch the edges of the wound together to stem the bleeding.* **2.** *Cover the area with gauze.*
3. *Support the embedded object with pads on either side.* **4.** *Bandage lightly over padding and secure.*

SPLINTERS

- Use a clean pair of tweezers to remove the splinter at the same angle that it entered the skin.
- If you cannot get at a splinter because it is under the skin, sterilize a needle and use it to gently lift the tip of the splinter. (Sterilize stainless steel needles or pins by holding the point over a burning match for a few seconds.)
- Wash the area and apply an adhesive dressing if necessary.
- If infection sets in, treat as appropriate.

BRUISING

- Limit swelling by immediately applying a cold compress to the injured area (if you don't have an ice pack, use a bag of frozen peas). If the bruise begins to throb, give a mild painkiller.
- Bruising under a finger- or toenail may result from a crush injury. Blood collects under the nail, turning it blue-black. If the blood is not drained out, the nail will usually fall off and be replaced by a new one. You can reduce the chance of the nail being lost by draining the blood painlessly as follows: heat one tip of a paperclip in a flame until it glows red-hot. Press the hot end of the paperclip gently on the middle of the blackened nail. When you feel the nail 'give', remove the paperclip and allow the blood to drain through the hole. Massage the nail gently to improve drainage.

PREVENTION

Many cuts, lacerations and penetration wounds can be avoided if care is taken when using knives, scissors, garden implements and workshop tools. Keep all sharp objects out of the reach of young children and, as soon as they are old enough to understand, teach them how to handle sharp-edged items.

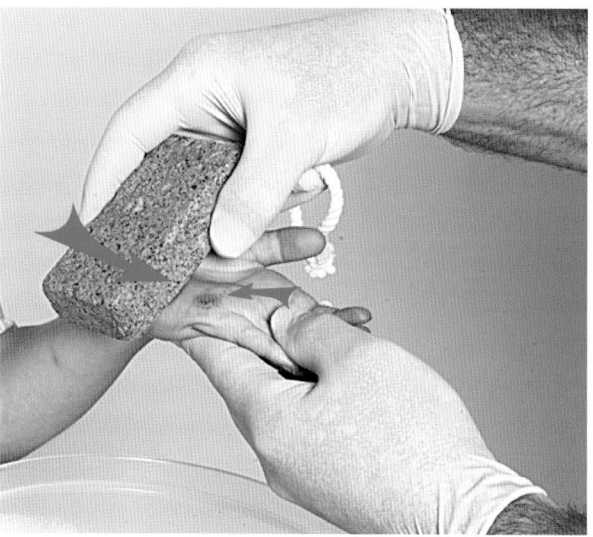

Use a pumice stone in the opposite direction the splinter entered to ease it out.

REMOVING A SPLINTER

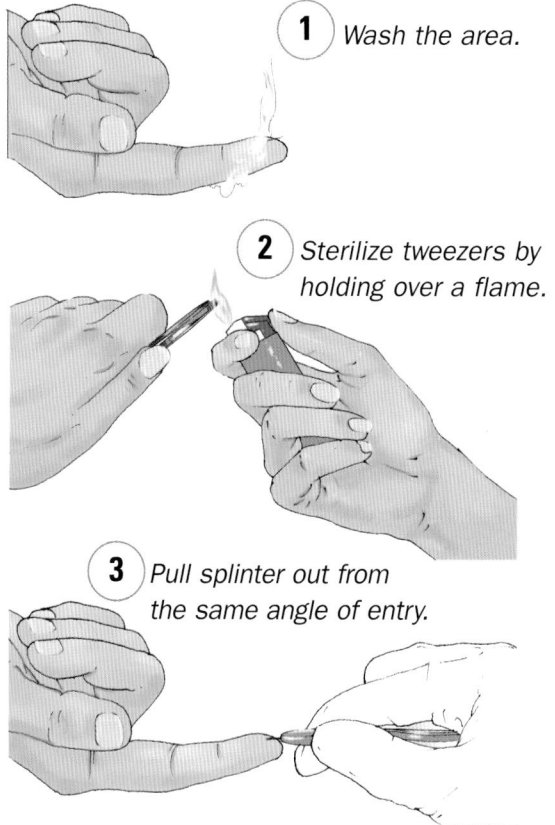

1 *Wash the area.*

2 *Sterilize tweezers by holding over a flame.*

3 *Pull splinter out from the same angle of entry.*

Bleeding from the mouth and nose

Because the mouth and nose are important sensory organs (taste and smell), both have an extremely rich blood supply. As a result, even small wounds inside the mouth or nose can bleed dramatically. Such injuries are most common in children, although nosebleeds can occur at all stages of life. Most injuries to the mouth and nose can be safely managed at home with the first-aid measures recommended below. Small injuries usually heal rapidly with minimal, if any, scarring, thanks to the excellent blood supply in these areas.

SYMPTOMS

- Bleeding due to any injury will usually be obvious within seconds, and accompanied by immediate pain.
- The site of bleeding from the mouth may be easy to confirm if the injury involves the lips, teeth and tongue, or gum margin. A small flashlight is useful for spotting injuries further back in the mouth cavity, such as puncture wounds caused by foreign objects.
- Blunt injuries may cause visible swelling of the injured area as well as bleeding.
- Spontaneous nosebleeds can occur at any time, but may be precipitated by sneezing, nose blowing or picking at dried secretions inside the nostril.

CAUSES

Bleeding from the mouth is common in children, usually a result of falls, or puncture wounds caused by solid objects e.g. pencils, ice cream or lollipop sticks carried in the mouth.

Children who are distracted while eating can accidentally bite into the tongue or lip, producing a painful, bleeding injury. The mouth and nose may be injured at any age by assault. Loosening or loss of a tooth will cause vigorous bleeding from the gum and tooth socket.

Spontaneous nosebleeds are common after colds and other viral infections which cause drying of the mucous lining, or as a consequence of repeated nose-blowing, or overuse of decongestant nasal sprays which interfere with normal mucus production.

PREVENTION

- Children should be discouraged from sucking on sharp or solid objects, and certainly from walking or running with such objects in their mouths.
- At mealtimes, children should be encouraged to eat slowly, and discouraged from speaking while chewing on solid food.
- Don't allow the inside of the nose to dry out, particularly after viral infections. If drying occurs, a twice-daily dab of petroleum jelly to each side of the septum will reduce the risk of nosebleeds.
- Limit use of decongestant nasal sprays to one or two days, if at all. Prolonged use dries out the nose and will also aggravate a blocked nose due to the 'rebound' effect of the medication.

TREATMENT

- Stem bleeding from the lips by applying a clean gauze pad soaked in iced water, and gently pinch the wound between your fingers. In a cooperative patient, the same technique can be used for small tongue injuries.
- Control bleeding in the mouth cavity by giving the casualty ice cubes to suck, or by rinsing and gargling with iced water. The water should be spat out, as swallowed blood may irritate the stomach and cause vomiting.
- Soak a lost tooth (or portion of a broken tooth) in milk or saltwater to preserve (so it can be reinserted by a dentist). A gauze swab soaked in very cold water can be pressed gently against the bleeding tooth socket.
- To stop a nosebleed, pinch together the soft part of the nostrils until bleeding ceases. While this constant pressure is being applied, hold the head slightly forward so that excess blood drips into the mouth and can be spat out.
- Persistent pain after injury can be treated with a mild painkiller.

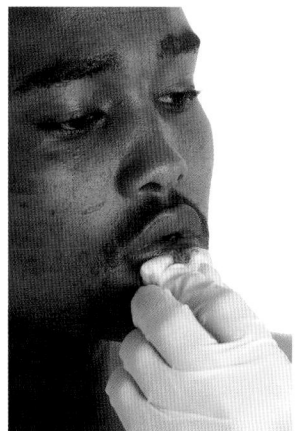

Pinch a lip wound together with a swab soaked in cold water.

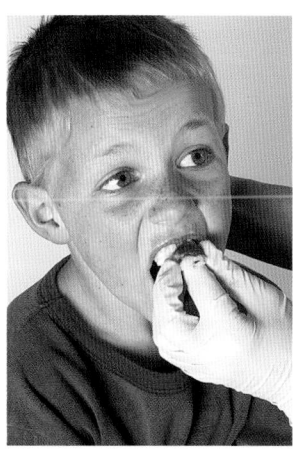

Hold a gauze swab against the tooth socket to stem the bleeding.

AFTERCARE

- Anyone with a mouth injury should avoid spicy or acidic foods for five days afterwards.
- Twice-daily teeth-brushing and rinsing the mouth after meals will reduce the risk of wound infection. If teeth or gums have been injured, twice-daily gargling with an antiseptic mouthwash can be done in place of teeth-brushing for the first few days.
- After blunt injury, the crooked appearance of a broken nose may only be obvious once the swelling settles down. If this happens, seek a medical opinion.

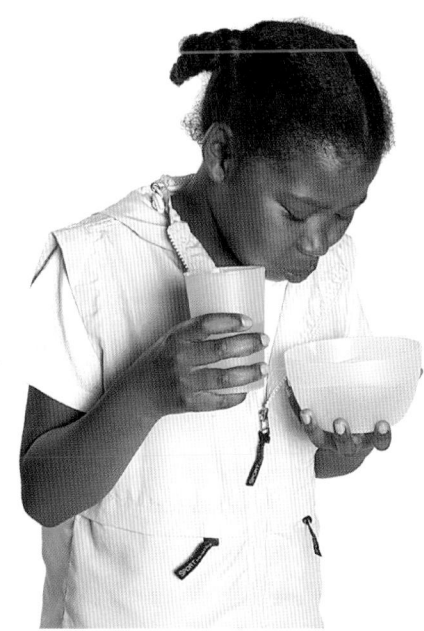

Rinse the injured mouth with water and antiseptic gargle, after every meal.

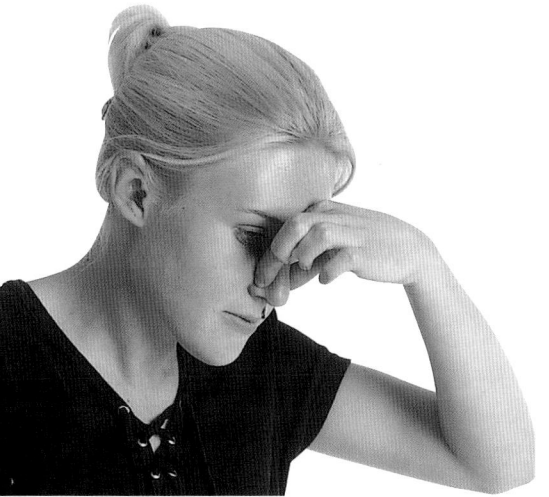

Gently pinching the nostrils will usually stop a nosebleed within 10 minutes.

Coughs, colds and croup

Upper respiratory tract infection (URTI) is an unfortunate part of life that most people have to endure at some time or other, particularly during the colder months, and certainly in countries that experience cold, wet winters. The incidence and severity of URTI are particularly higher in smokers.Most 'common' colds are mild, self-limiting and require nothing more than symptomatic treatment. However, the risk of complications and related illness may be greater in babies, infants, elderly people, and anyone with chronic lung disease, or other illnesses or conditions that interfere with the body's normal immune response to infection.

SYMPTOMS

- Common colds typically present with mild fever, cough, nasal discharge and persistent sneezing, with or without a sore throat. Fever is more marked in infants and children than in adults. Muscle aches, high fever and chills are more typical of influenza than a common cold.
- Cough, due to post-nasal drip following an URTI, may be accompanied by a sore throat, an offensive taste in the mouth, and yellow-green sputum produced by coughing.
- The typical 'wheeze' (prolonged exhalation of air) differentiates a bout of asthma from URTI. (*See* **asthma** p100).
- Prolonged fits of coughing followed by a 'whoop' as a child struggles for breath, typify whooping cough. Symptoms may persist for up to three months and can recur.
- Croup presents as a barking or crowing sound when a child coughs. It is usually worst at night.

CAUSES

- Most URTI are caused by viruses, although bacteria may prolong or aggravate an existing illness.
- Chronic sinus infection causes post-nasal drip, where infected secretions leak into the windpipe and lungs, resulting in a persistent cough, with or without mild fever.
- When coughing is a dominant symptom, it may be difficult to distinguish URTI from asthma, although the two conditions do co-exist, often in children.
- The bacterium *Bordetella pertussis* causes whooping cough (*see* **common childhood infections** p92) which can be prevented by immunization.
- Croup describes the typical barking cough heard in children between six months and three years of age. It is most commonly caused by a viral infection involving the area just below the larynx (voice box). A severe form of croup is caused by *Haemophilus influenza*, a bacterium which causes swelling of the epiglottis (epiglottitis), leading to high fever, drooling saliva and difficulty with swallowing foods.
- An isolated cough may have many non-infectious causes, including the side-effects of medication, such as drugs used to control blood pressure, foreign bodies impacted in the respiratory tract, lung tumours or tumours elsewhere in the chest.
- Suspect an inhaled foreign body in a child with chronic cough, shortness of breath and fever, particularly if a course of antibiotics has been given without success.

TREATMENT

- **Common colds may be safely treated at home**. Rest, drink plenty of fluids and take paracetamol or aspirin to bring down fever. That is usually all that is necessary. Medicated lozenges are ineffective against viruses and are no better than warm drinks and glucose or boiled sweets for soothing a sore throat.
- Like aches and pains, **a cough is a warning symptom, not a diagnosis**. It serves to expel infected secretions or other harmful agents from the respiratory tract. Therefore, medication which suppresses the cough reflex may do more harm than good, and is not recommended as first-line treatment for adults or children. The priority is to identify and treat the cause, not just the symptom.
- Both **whooping cough and viral croup** may be treated at home, but always in consultation with your doctor, in case complications arise.

 SEEK MEDICAL HELP IF:

- cold symptoms do not clear up within three to four days, or become worse, suggesting bacterial infection.
- there is a cough or a breathing difficulty (with or without fever) in a child under six months of age.
- symptoms are suggestive of asthma.
- symptoms are suggestive of either whooping cough or croup.
- a cough persists even after the other cold symptoms have disappeared.
- a cough produces infected-looking sputum or blood.
- persistent dry coughing occurs as an isolated symptom.

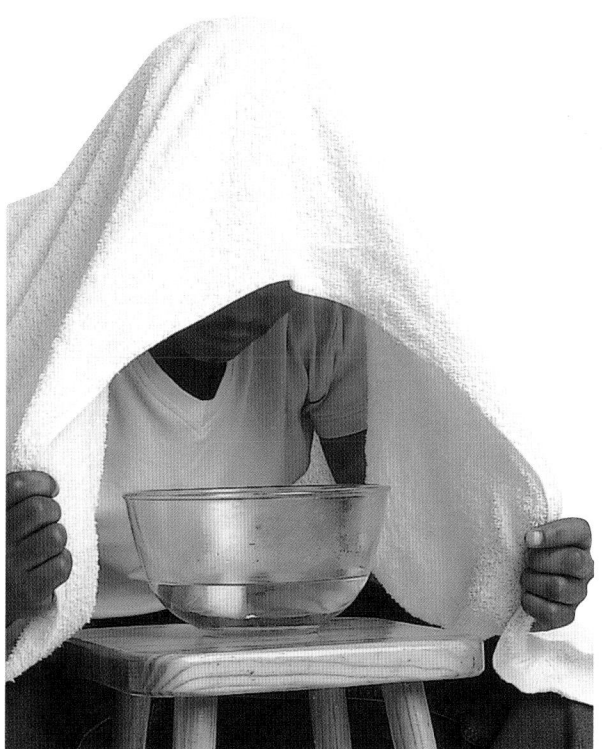

Inhaling steamy vapours can help clear a blocked nose and relieve congestion.

PREVENTION

- You can reduce the risk of colds and other viral infections by protecting your immune system, particularly during the colder months of the year. Avoiding overexertion or stress, maintaining a healthy balanced diet, and ensuring that you are protected against extreme temperatures does not guarantee you won't contract viral infection, but certainly makes it less likely.
- Do not smoke! However many (or few) cigarettes you smoke each day, your risk of respiratory infection and many other diseases, will be greater than the average non-smoker.
- Ensure that your child is immunized against the bacteria which cause whooping cough and epiglottitis (*Haemophilus* influenza).
- Keep small objects such as toy parts, coins, pins, clips and bits of jewellery away from infants and toddlers. Peanuts should not be given to children under the age of five years, due to the risks of choking and aspiration into the lung.

Common childhood infections

Infections caused by viruses and occasionally bacteria, are common in younger children. Most of these infections are picked up from infected siblings or other children, and the risk increases significantly as soon as children begin to mix freely at crèches, playschool or in similar social settings. Most childhood infections are mild, and even beneficial, as each exposure stimulates and strengthens the child's developing immune system. Although most childhood infections can be safely treated at home, it is advisable to notify your regular doctor or clinic if your child develops any of the infections listed on the following pages.

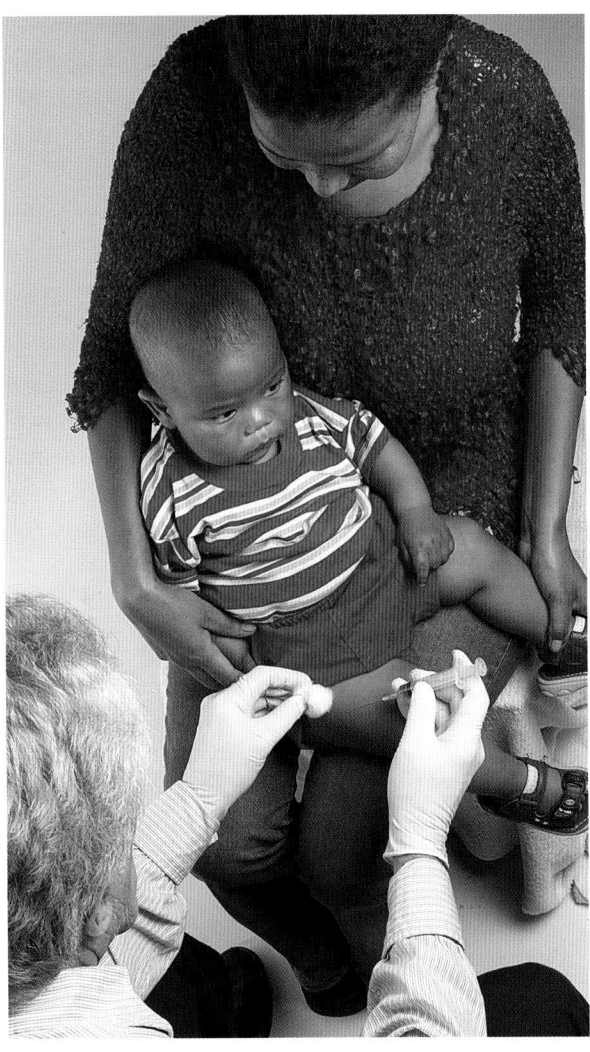

CAUSES

Viruses cause the majority of common childhood infections. Bacterial infection is less common and, once recognized, can be successfully treated with prescribed antibiotics.

Fortunately, routine immunization schedules protect most children against measles, rubella (German measles), mumps, diphtheria, tuberculosis (TB), whooping cough, polio and viral hepatitis, which would otherwise threaten the lives of thousands of children each year.

Nevertheless, these infections do still occur occasionally, as do others such as chicken pox and infectious mononucleosis (glandular fever) which are not covered by immunization.

PREVENTION

- Ensure your child's immunizations are up to date. If in any doubt, consult your doctor or clinic.
- Children with any chronic illness or depressed immunity, should be shielded as far as possible from contact with people known to be infected with viruses or bacteria.
- Women in the first trimester (three months) of pregnancy should not be exposed to anyone possibly infected with the rubella virus.

Keep up to date with your child's immunizations.

ILLNESSES AND SYMPTOMS

Virtually all common childhood infections are characterized by general, nonspecific symptoms, followed sooner or later by the appearance of a skin rash and/or other local signs, such as gland enlargement.

CHICKEN POX

Most children get chicken pox at some time. It is highly contagious and spreads easily. Mild fever and headache are followed, within hours, by clusters of pimples on the trunk that often spread to the face and scalp and sometimes inside the mouth. The pimples change into itchy blisters that dry within days. The scabs that can remain itchy for some time.

The only complication of note is secondary bacterial infection of the blisters, caused by scratching. Pneumonia and encephalitis are rare complications.

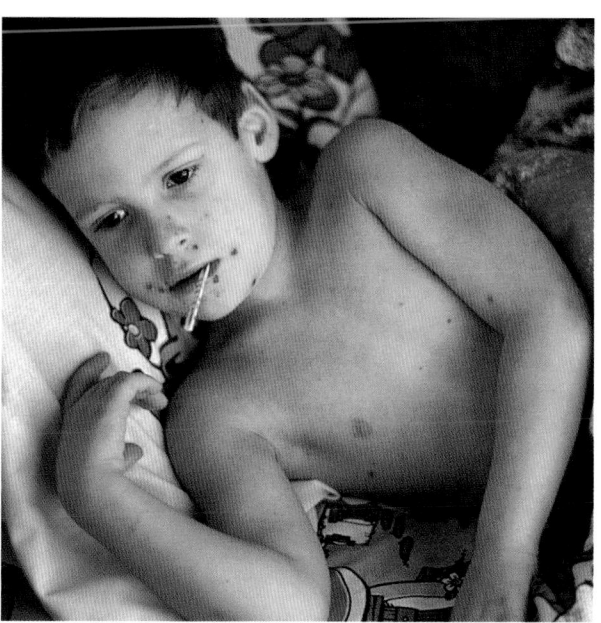

A four-year-old boy with chicken pox.

ERYTHEMA INFECTIOSUM

This common infection usually occurs in children older than two years and is sometimes referred to as 'slapped cheek disease'. Mild fever and bright red discoloration of the cheeks are followed after a few days by a pink blotchy rash on the arms, legs, and sometimes, the body. It may take 4–6 weeks for the rash to disappear entirely, but the child will feel better long before this. Complications are rare.

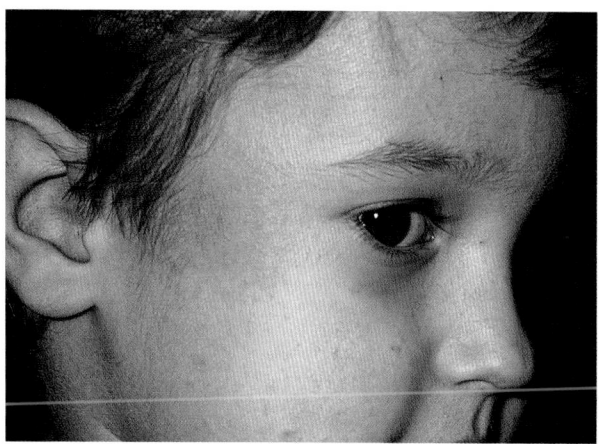

Slapped cheek disease.

GLANDULAR FEVER

This disease is most common in older children and young adults. High fever, often associated with fatigue, poor appetite, sore throat and headache may persist for days or weeks. Lymph glands in the neck and elsewhere may become swollen and tender. Full recovery may take a few weeks.

MEASLES

Fever, dry cough and inflammation of the eyes and nose are followed after four to five days by the appearance of a flat, red blotchy skin rash on the

 CAUTION

If you suspect **measles**, report to your doctor.

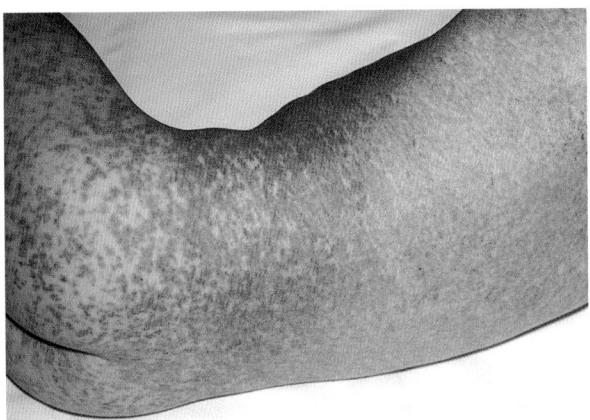

Measles

MUMPS

Mild fever and discomfort around the lower face are followed within a day or two by painful swelling of the salivary glands on one or both sides of the face. The swelling usually goes within a week or so. In some children, the infection may spread, causing inflammation of the brain, pancreas or (in boys) testes. Most children recover fully within 10–12 days.

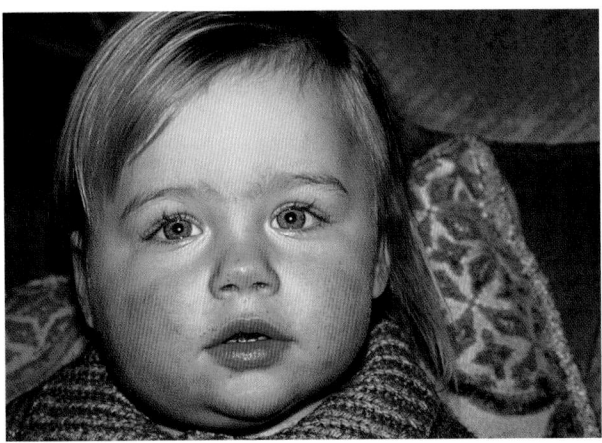

Mumps

face, gradually spreading to the rest of the body. The rash usually clears up within a week, by which time the child feels better. Possible complications include diarrhoea, middle ear infection, pneumonia and encephalitis (spread of the infection to the brain), but these are most likely to occur in infancy and in children suffering from malnutrition or other chronic health problems.

RUBELLA (GERMAN MEASLES)

Rubella is a milder infection than measles and may sometimes pass unnoticed, or be misdiagnosed as flu. Mild fever and swelling of the lymph glands behind the ears and at the back of the neck are typically followed after a day or two by a rash of tiny pink spots beginning on the face and then spreading to the rest of the body. The rash seldom lasts longer than three to four days. Some children may develop pain in their joints, but other complications are rare. The illness usually resolves within 10 days.

The greatest danger from rubella is to women in the early stages of pregnancy, as the virus may cause severe harm to the developing foetus.

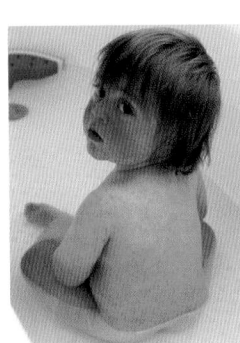

Rubella

ROSEOLA INFANTUM

This is common viral infection in children before the age of two. A sudden high fever may be accompanied by diarrhoea, cough and swollen neck glands. After three to four days the temperature begins to drop and light pink spots appear on the head, neck and body. By the time they disappear within four to five days the child should have recovered. Complications are rare in healthy children.

 CAUTION

A child with **rubella** must not have contact with a pregnant woman, especially during her first three months of pregnancy.

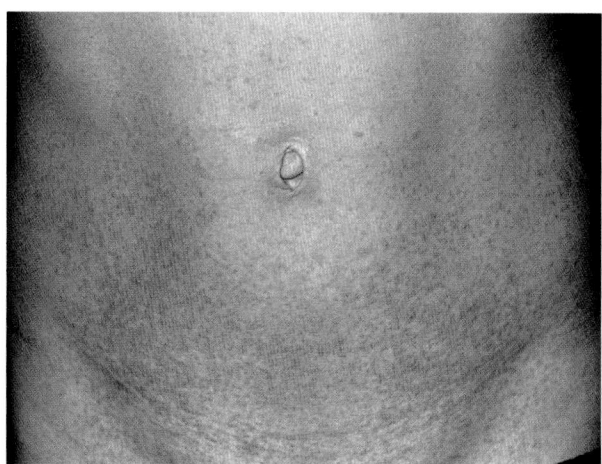
Scarlet fever

SCARLET FEVER

This bacterial infection is less common nowadays due to the availability of antibiotics. Initially, fever, sore throat and headache are common, sometimes accompanied by nausea and vomiting. Within 12 hours, a red rash appears on the neck and chest, spreading to the rest of the body. The face appears flushed, but the area around the mouth is spared. The tonsils may be enlarged. A white coating appears on the tongue, but peels off after a few days, leaving a strawberry red appearance, due to prominently raised, red taste buds. After a few days, skin affected by the rash may begin to peel.

Complications are rare, provided the diagnosis is promptly confirmed, and antibiotics are commenced without delay.

WHOOPING COUGH

This is a highly contagious bacterial infection, which has become much less common thanks to immunization. For the first seven to 10 days, there may be a mild fever and dry cough which is troublesome mainly at night. Thereafter, the cough becomes more persistent, occurring in prolonged spasms followed by a gasp for breath, which produces the characteristic 'whoop' sound.

Vomiting or seizures may follow coughing attacks. This second stage of the illness may last for up to three months, and the symptoms can recur if the child develops another respiratory tract infection. Infants with whooping cough may become quite exhausted by the persistent coughing.

MENINGITIS (*SEE ALSO* PP46–7)

Meningitis is not usually grouped with the common childhood infections, but can occur in mini-epidemics, particularly where large numbers of children live in close contact, as in boarding schools.

Meningitis is the inflammation of the tissues lining the brain, usually as a result of viral or bacterial infection. **Viral meningitis** is the milder variety, while **bacterial meningitis** can be life threatening. Both may present as a flu-like illness with fever, loss of appetite, headache and irritability. Neck stiffness, or resistance to movement of the neck usually aids diagnosis (difficult in infants and toddlers). Tiny blood spots under the skin, and sometimes larger areas of fresh bruising are typical of a severe variety caused by *Neisseria meningitidis*.

Meningitis is a life-threatening condition that requires immediate medical attention, including antibiotics and life-support measures (see pp46–7)

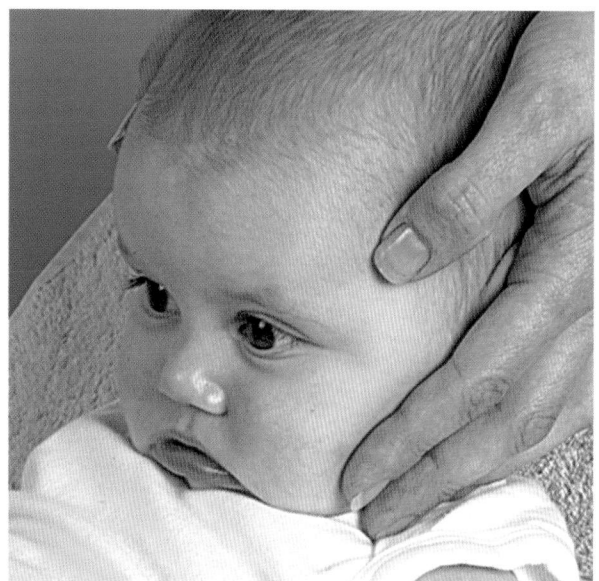
Meningitis causes a stiff neck that cannot be flexed without discomfort. Steady the chest with one hand and place the other behind the child's head, pushing down gently.

TREATMENT OF CHILDHOOD ILLNESSES

GENERAL SYMPTOMS

A high fever may be brought down successfully by sponging the child with tepid water, dressing them as cool as possible and administering medication such as paracetamol/acetaminophen. Aspirin may only be given to older children.

When they are feverish, children tend not to have much appetite for food. Don't make them more miserable by insisting that they should eat, but do encourage them to drink frequently in order to prevent dehydration.

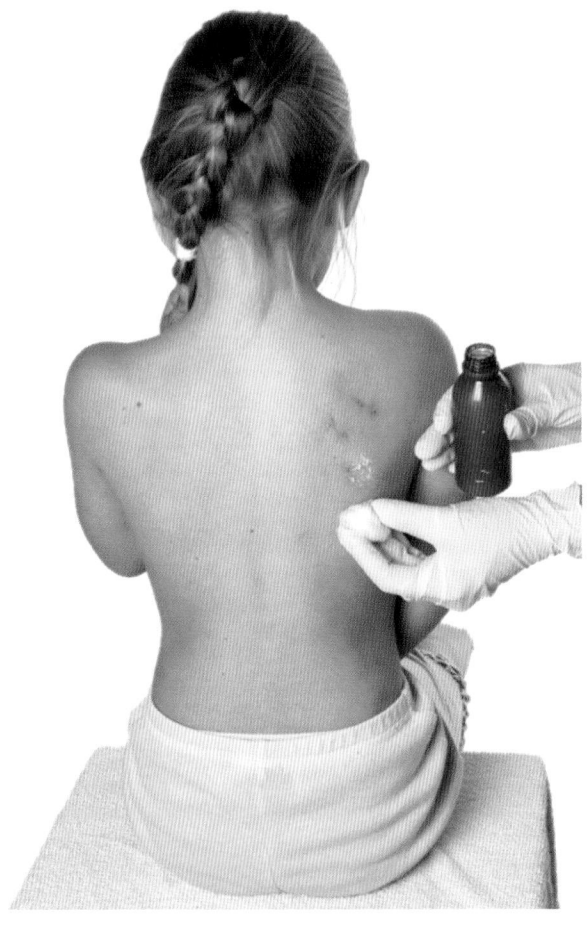

Calamine lotion helps to soothe the itch, and dry out the spots on the skin caused by infections such as chicken pox.

Cough suppressant medication should never be administered unless it has been prescribed especially for the child by a doctor.

Vomiting and diarrhoea usually resolve on their own and do not require specific treatment.

SKIN RASHES

Most skin rashes require no specific treatment. The itchy blisters of chicken pox can be treated with twice-daily application of calamine lotion, and antihistamine medication. Every effort should be taken

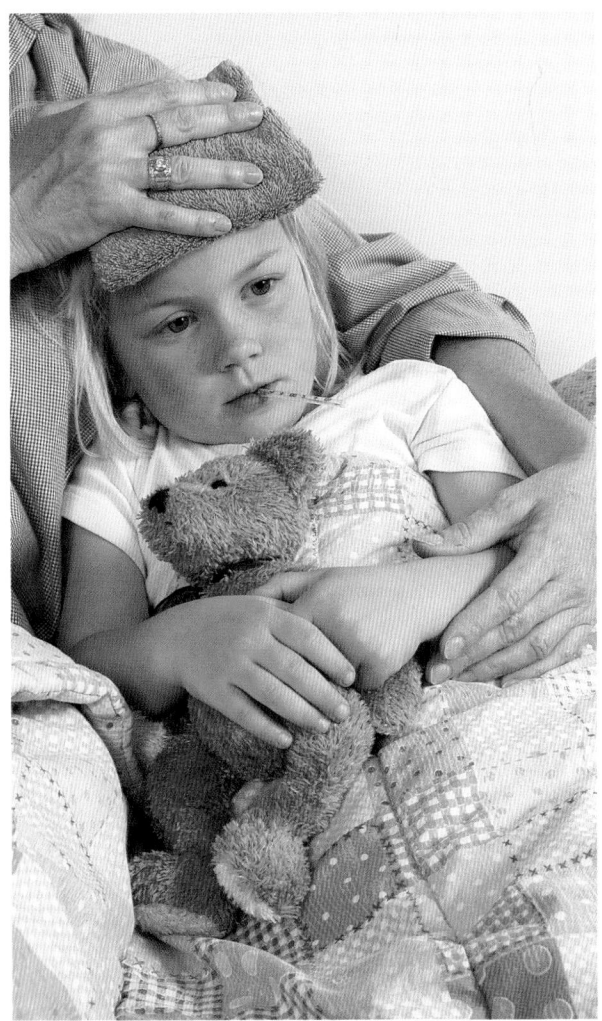

First take the child's temperature.

to discourage the child from scratching the blisters or scabs, as this may lead to secondary infection and even permanent scarring.

TREATING THE INFECTING AGENT

Antibiotics are only required for bacterial infections, and are of no value in uncomplicated viral infections.

TIP

Avoid infecting others: Keep a child with any of the infections listed on pp92–95 at home until your doctor considers him no longer infectious. Wash your hands well after each physical contact, as this will reduce the risk of transmission to other family members.

SEEK MEDICAL HELP IF:

- The child has a known chronic illness
- You are unsure of the symptoms and find it difficult to diagnose with precision.
- An infant who is under six months of age, develops one of the infections listed on pp92–95.
- A high fever fails to respond to your home treatment.
- The child appears exhausted, listless, or even too tired to breathe.
- The child becomes drowsy.
- The child has seizures.
- A baby vomits up all of its feeds.
- A child becomes ill again after an initial period of recovery.
- There is neck stiffness, blood spots or bruising (*see* **meningitis**, pp46–7).

The very best treatment for most childhood illnesses is bed rest and quiet, lots of love and attention and a tight hug from the favourite teddy.

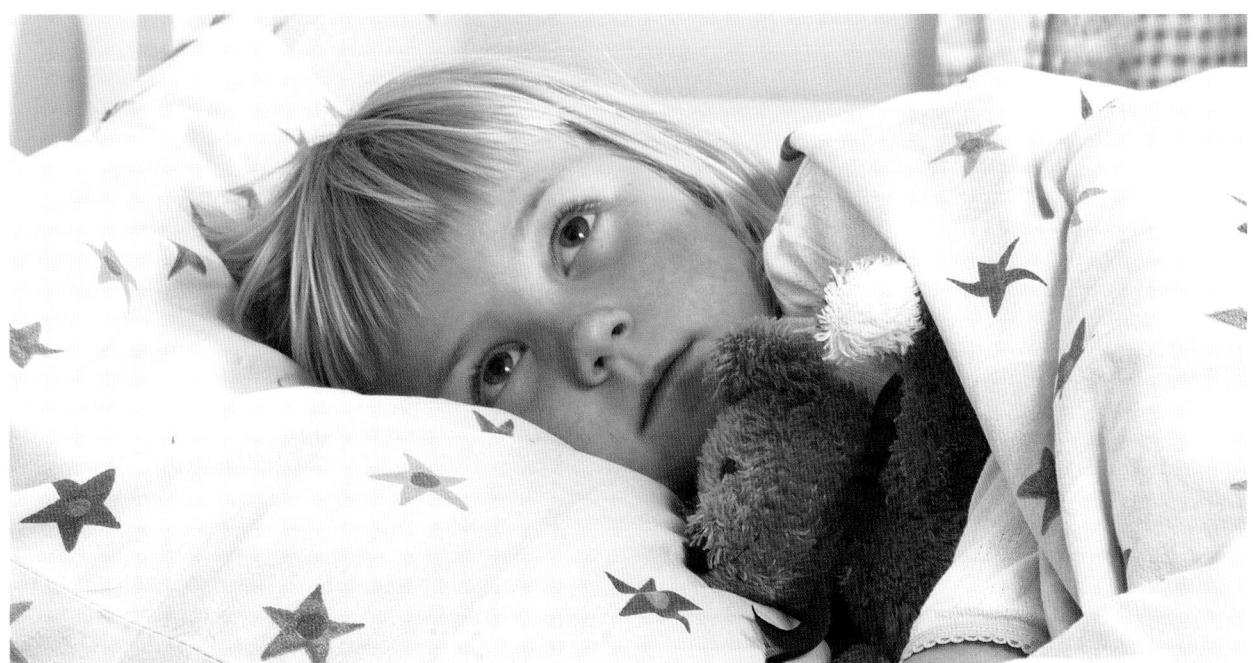

Headaches and migraines

Although millions of people worldwide suffer from headaches, most attacks are mild and do not require medical attention. Primary headaches are those which have no specific cause, but may be triggered by certain stimuli. Tension headache is by far the most common variety of primary headache, particularly in women. Cluster headaches, which are less common, but extremely painful, occur more frequently in men. Secondary headaches may be a symptom of a serious underlying illness or injury, where treatment is aimed at the cause, rather than the symptom. Migraine is a syndrome, of which headache is a common feature. However, the treatment and prevention of migraine are similar to that for other primary headaches.

SYMPTOMS

- Tension headache is a mild to moderate ache, or a band of pressure affecting both sides of the head and is often felt behind the eyes, with or without tension in the neck muscles. It may last a few hours, or build gradually during the day. It almost always comes on during daytime and seldom affects sleep. Most sufferers have one to two tension headaches per month.
- Cluster headaches typically strike with distressing frequency over a period of weeks, then disappear for months before returning. They can occur several times a day – often at night. They begin without warning and are agonizingly painful, but seldom last longer than an hour. They are usually felt on one side of the head, although not always the same side. The eye on the side of the pain often becomes inflamed and watery and the nostril may be blocked.

CAUSES

Many things can trigger primary headaches and avoiding these can do much to stop a headache from occurring in the first place.

Common triggers include stress, depression, fatigue, nicotine, caffeine, foods like ice cream, eye strain, hormonal variations due to menstruation, and some medications. Chronic use of painkillers for headache may precipitate withdrawal headaches. Alcohol often triggers cluster headaches.

Secondary headache may be a symptom of infection, head injury, disorders of the blood circulation, brain tumours, or chronic illnesses such as diabetes.

Mild headaches commonly occur in the early stages of viral and other infections.

Migraine is thought to result from the liberation of a chemical known as serotonin around blood vessels in and around the brain. Migraine attacks vary in severity from person to person and are typically preceded by warning symptoms such as mood changes, tingling sensations or visual images like zig-zag lines or flashing lights. The headache is usually one-sided, and may be accompanied by nausea and vomiting.

Migraines seldom last more than an hour, but a feeling of exhaustion or general illness may persist for longer. In children, migraine may present as abdominal pain with no headache.

TREATMENT

Wherever possible, trigger factors should be identified and avoided (*see* Prevention).

· Tension headache and mild migraine usually respond well to mild painkillers such as asprin or paracetamol/acetaminophen, and these should always be the first treatment option. Non-steroidal anti-inflammatory drugs may be helpful for some people, but should only be used after consultation with a doctor.

· Cluster headaches usually require prescription drugs, many of them not specifically intended for this purpose. Always seek a medical opinion if you suspect that you may be suffering from cluster headaches.

· The duration of all headaches may be limited by rest and relaxation until the pain wears off.

PREVENTION

The key to reducing primary headaches is recognizing and avoiding the trigger factors.

· If your headaches recur frequently, keep a diary to record and identify possible trigger factors.

CAUTION

● Secondary headache can occur at any age. It occurs 'out of the blue' in someone not normally prone to headache

● A headache following head or facial trauma requires urgent medical attention

● A headache associated with fever, persistent nausea or vomiting, drowsiness, lossed or blurred vision, convulsions, speech disorders, muscle weakness or abnormal behaviour, could indicate a serious underlying disorder and requires medical attention.

· If you suffer from cluster headaches, avoid alcohol during attacks, and limit your intake during attack-free intervals.

· Headaches experienced while in any static position may be related to bad posture or muscle strain. Consult a physiotherapist or occupational therapist.

· Headaches accompanied by burning or itching eyes, particularly while reading or working at a computer, suggest eye-strain or visual disorders, and require the opinion of an optometrist.

· If you take regular medication for a chronic condition, ask your doctor whether headache is a possible side-effect of the medication.

· Your doctor may prescribe drugs to reduce the frequency of cluster headaches or migraine, if attacks are frequent enough to interfere with your lifestyle.

· If you suffer frequent headaches, be careful about increasing your pain-relief medication, as overuse can cause withdrawal headaches. Consult a doctor about alternative methods of pain relief or headache prevention.

SEEK MEDICAL HELP IF:

● If headaches cause persistent pain for more than 15 days each month.

● If headaches persist for more than 24 hours without relief.

● Mild painkillers don't help.

● You suspect a cluster headache.

● There are symptoms which suggest a secondary headache (*see* above).

● If the patient is a child, and if the headache is associated with fever, drowsiness and/or the appearance of purplish spots on the body. These may indicate meningitis and require immediate investigation and treatment.

Asthma

Asthma is a disease in which the airways become narrowed as a result of inflammation, reducing airflow and causing the wheezing, coughing, shortness of breath and tight chest which one normally associates with this condition. It is also known as bronchial asthma, exercise-induced asthma, or reactive airways disease (RAD). Asthma is incurable, but ongoing treatment and self-discipline can enable sufferers to lead a normal life. Treatment involves long-term medications which are used on a regular basis to combat the condition, plus quick-relief measures to combat an attack. In children, the condition may improve or disappear as they grow older.

SYMPTOMS

Asthma attacks usually begin suddenly.
Symptoms include:

- Breathing that requires greater effort
- Shortness of breath aggravated by exercise
- Tight chest
- Wheezing or coughing with or without the production of sputum (phlegm)
- Abnormal, laboured breathing pattern in which breathing out takes more than twice as long as breathing in

CAUSES

- Air pollutants such as wind-borne dust or cigarette smoke
- Animal hair and skin flakes (dander)
- Bee stings (also bites or stings from other insects)
- Cold air
- Dust mites
- Exercise
- Foods, especially nuts and shellfish
- Emotional stress
- Medications
- Moulds
- Plants and pollens

TREATMENT

If an asthma sufferer has an attack, get them their medication and help to administer it; calm them and give them space and air. In the case of a first-time attack, or if they don't have an inhaler with them, and they continue having difficulty breathing, call for assistance.

PREVENTION

Sufferers, particularly children, should use their medication before exercise to prevent attacks. Sufferers should try to minimize their exposure to factors that can trigger attacks. Many of the principles apply for asthma as for the prevention of **allergies** (see p101).

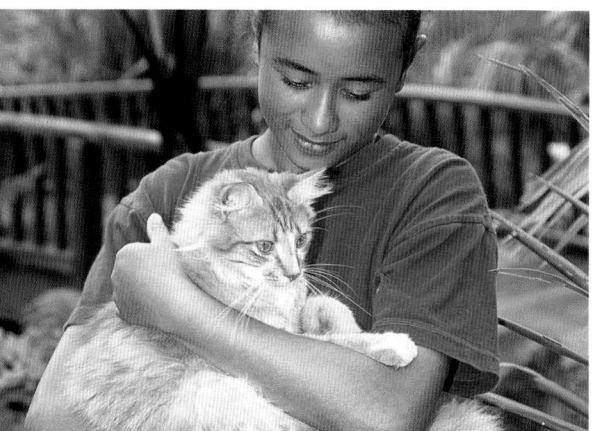

Above: *Animal hair and skin flakes can trigger allergic reactions in susceptible individuals.*
Right: *Asthma sufferers usually carry an inhaler to help relieve symptoms.*

Allergies

Most people with hay fever and other outdoor allergies think of their home as a haven where they can escape their allergies. Wrong! Houses and apartment buildings harbour and trap their own allergens, making them impossible to avoid. An allergic reaction is a response by your body's immune system to a foreign invader (a substance, such as dust or pollen, that is not native to your body). Exposure to this invader, or allergen, triggers the allergic reaction. Reactions to allergens vary from mild to severe. They might appear immediately on exposure to an allergen or after repeated exposure.

When the immune system becomes sensitized to a specific invader, it overreacts to it. This overreaction to an often-harmless substance is known as a hypersensitivity reaction and sets in motion the release of chemicals, or mediators, such as histamine. It is the effect of the mediators on cells and tissues that causes the symptoms of an allergic reaction. Severe allergic reaction, or anaphylaxis, is rare but can be life threatening, as it causes shock and narrowing of the airways, making breathing difficult.

SYMPTOMS

The symptoms of indoor allergic reactions are those of many other allergic reactions:
- Watery nasal discharge
- Sneezing
- Itchy, stuffy nose (see also p90)
- Itchy, watery, swollen or bloodshot eyes
- Scratchy, swollen throat
- Difficulty in breathing
- Tightness in the chest or throat
- Unexplained wheezing or shortness of breath
- Rapid or irregular heartbeat
- Hives (also known as urticaria or nettle rash), is the formation of itchy red or white raised patches on the skin

CAUSES

Pet dander (skin particles): Contrary to popular belief, an allergic reaction to an animal is not caused by hair or fur, but by substances in dander (dead skin flakes) that become loosened from the animal's skin when it licks or scratches itself. The allergens are released into the air, where they join the other components of house dust. Furred or feathered animals, such as cats, dogs, hamsters and birds, are most likely to cause allergic reactions, which may be triggered by the following:
- Playing with the animal, especially indoors.
- Cleaning animal beds, cages, or litter boxes.
- Exposure to furniture, carpets, bedding, clothing, animal beds or cages, and pet's toys where allergens might be present.
- Being in an indoor area with another person whose clothes carry the allergens.

Moulds: Moulds, a type of fungus that is generally found outdoors, are a common trigger of hay fever symptoms, as their method of reproduction results in millions of spores being released into the air. Being so tiny, moulds are impossible to keep out of a home and there is virtually no surface on which they will not thrive. All mould needs is water, or even just humidity greater than 50 per cent, hence the proliferation of mildew (a type of mould) in showers, bathrooms or any poorly ventilated space.

Cockroaches: 'Roaches' are a fact of life in homes all over the world and although they are not a major source of allergens while alive (apart from their waste when it dries), when they die their remains dry and disintegrate, adding to the house dust.

Foods: Genuine food allergies, which affect the immune system, should not be confused with food intolerance, which affects the digestive system. One of the most widespread food allergies is to nuts, especially peanuts (groundnuts). Other foods which can cause a severe allergic reaction include are seafood, eggs and strawberries. Many children are allergic to cow's milk, and wheat or wheat-based products can cause a condition known as coeliac disease.

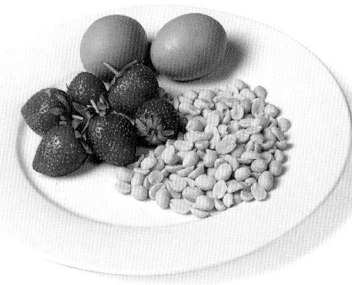

Strawberries, eggs and nuts are common allergy triggers.

TWO COMMON MANIFESTATIONS

Allergic rhinitis (hay fever), an inflammation of the membranes lining the nose and throat, occurs when airborne substances (allergens) are inhaled and come to rest in the linings of the eyes, nose or airway of a susceptible person. Allergic rhinitis can be perennial (occuring all year round) as a result of house dust, dust mites, animal dander, feathers or mould spores. Seasonal allergic rhinitis is caused by grass, tree or flower pollens. It occurs mostly during spring and summer, when pollen counts are high, hence the common name, hay fever.

Urticaria, also known as hives, is an itchy rash that results from exposure to a variety of allergens,

SEEK MEDICAL HELP IF:

In some cases, a severe reaction to certain foods can cause **anaphylactic shock** (*see* p40), leading to difficulty in breathing, dizziness, or loss of consciousness. **This is a medical emergency and requires immediate attention.** If your symptoms suggest an anaphylactic reaction, get to an emergency room immediately. Do not drive yourself, as the symptoms may become more pronounced en route and you could have an accident.

Symptoms include:
- Tightness in the chest or throat
- Difficulty in breathing
- Dizziness, light-headedness or fainting
- Loss of consciousness
- Hives (*see* symptoms below)

including food, insect bites and plants. The raised, red rash of acute urticaria usually disappears within a few hours, but chronic urticaria can persist for days or weeks and both forms can recur.

TREATMENT

Seek medical attention if the symptoms become more pronounced over a day or two, or if they fail to improve after the source of the allergen has been removed. The elimination of an allergen is obviously the best course of remedy. Unfortunately, when it comes to house dust, the best you can do is to limit the amount of dust with a suitable housekeeping routine, and treat the symptoms.

If your symptoms do not improve, your health-care provider may prescribe one or more medications, either for the treatment of an allergic 'attack' or as a prophylactic (preventative medication), to dampen the allergic response.

Self-care at home: Antihistamine medications can be taken to reduce itching and watery eyes. Some are long-acting and can be taken over the long-term.

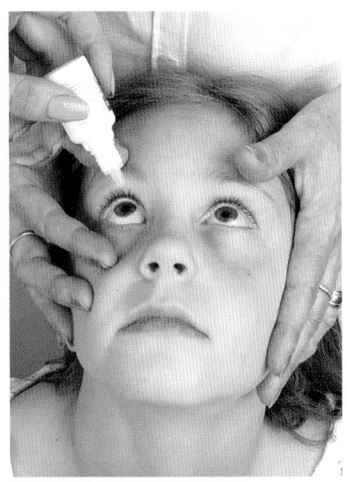

Decongestant eye-drops help to soothe itchy eyes.

Certain antihistamines may make you too drowsy to drive or operate machinery safely. In the case of children, their schoolwork may be affected, but the effects of the sedation can be reduced by using slow-release antihistamines.

Calamine lotion is useful for treating urticaria (hives) and decongestant eye drops help to soothe scratchy eyes. Nasal decongestants are to be used sparingly as there is a risk of a rebound effect if they are used too often or for longer than 24 hours.

Remedial therapy: In cases where a single allergen can be identified as the trigger for allergic rhinitis, the doctor may prescribe a course of injections that will result in desensitizing the patient over a period of time (immunotherapy). Severe seasonal rhinitis can be relieved by nasal spray and eye drops containing cromolyn sodium. Topical steroid nasal sprays are also effective.

PREVENTION

The single best thing you can do to stop the reaction is to reduce your exposure to the allergens. In the case of a much-loved family pet, the choice can be a very difficult one – to keep it or get rid of it. In any event, it can take months for the symptoms to disappear. An alternative is to keep the pet outdoors and/or have another member of the family take care of it so that your contact is reduced as much as possible.

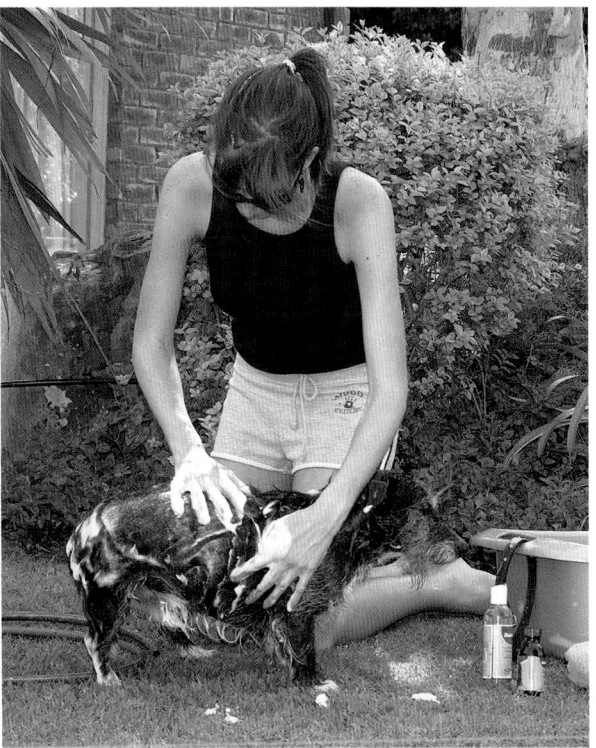

If anyone in your household suffers from allergies: regular grooming may help to reduce your pet's hair loss and thus prevent an allergic reaction.

Regular, frequent grooming of the pet might also help, but beware of causing skin problems which can actually exacerbate the problem. It helps to avoid long-haired animals, as they tend to shed greater quantities of hair than short-haired cats and dogs.

Fabric surfaces are ideal temporary traps for small particles so the fewer carpets, curtains, drapes and cloth-upholstered chairs you have, the better. Where possible, substitute tiles or wood for carpeting, fabric upholstery with leather and curtains with blinds. Ensure surfaces are kept clean and dust-free and that bedding and clothing are laundered regularly. Your pet's bedding should also be washed frequently and aired in the sun whenever possible.

Deal with mould and mildew by ensuring good ventilation in bathrooms and kitchens. Mould on ceilings can be kept in check by wiping with dilute bleach (sodium hypochloride) or using paint impregnated with fungicide.

Bites and stings

Bite injuries can be divided into those that affect mainly the skin and soft tissues (such as those from a dog, a cat and human bites) and those where there is an injection of venom or poison (from spiders, snakes and marine creatures). In the case of animal-inflicted injuries, the risk of infection is often more of a concern than the damage caused by the bite. Human bites should always be treated as an emergency, however minor they might seem. Non-venomous insect bites are usually harmless, causing local discomfort, itching and swelling, but the venom injected by some insects and the bites of certain snakes and spiders can cause a systemic reaction (affecting the whole body), which may require life support and antivenom.

 SEEK MEDICAL HELP IF:

- there are breathing difficulties. Check **ABC** (*see* pp22–3 and p165); start life support; continue until medical help arrives (*see* **rescue breathing** p26; **anaphylactic shock**, p42).
- the casualty has been seriously bitten, particularly if the attack involved a wild or unknown animal.
- the wound needs stitches. (Especially facial and hand wounds require urgent medical attention.)
- the casualty has not had a tetanus shot in the last five years.
- any bite has broken the skin.

ANIMAL BITES

With animal-inflicted bites, the skin is usually broken and bleeding, and there may be puncture wounds, crush injuries and/or bruising. Minor bites can be treated with thorough washing, cleaning and dressing with a dab of antiseptic ointment, but all bites on the hand or face require medical attention. Cat bites carry a higher risk of infection than dog bites. Unless you have recently had a tetanus shot, you should get one within 24 hours of any skin break.

 DO NOT

- let a snake bite-victim move around. Keep them still to prevent the spread of venom and, if necessary, carry them to safety.
- apply a tourniquet or other constricting device over a snake bite, or attempt to cut the wound or apply any form of suction to 'remove' the poison.

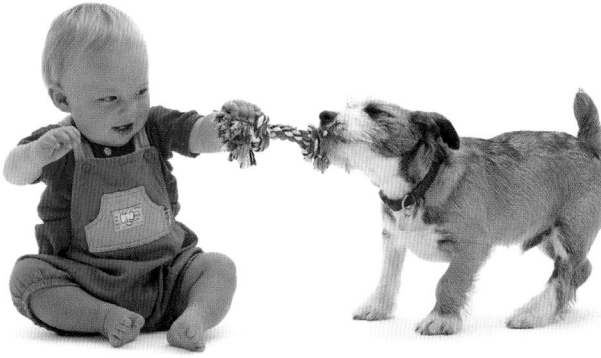

Sharp canine teeth can inflict a painful wound on a child's delicate skin, so don't let play become too boisterous.

BITE INJURIES

CAUSES

Pets are the most common cause of animal bites. Children are most at risk, and the decision to keep pets when there are toddlers in the home must be carefully taken.

Cage birds, too, can inflict a nasty bite, so children should be discouraged from sticking their fingers through the bars.

PREVENTION

- Teach your children to treat animals with respect, and not to tease or provoke them.
- Do not approach strange animals, and teach your children not to do so either.
- Choose pets carefully, particularly if you have small children, and buy from a reputable breeder. Females are less aggressive than males; some breeds are more tolerant than others.

TREATMENT FOR ANIMAL AND HUMAN BITES

- Calm and reassure the casualty.
- To prevent contamination, wear latex gloves, and wash your hands thoroughly with soap before and after attending to any wound.
- Wash the wound thoroughly using mild soap and running water. Cover with antiseptic ointment and bandage with clean dressing.
- If the bite is bleeding heavily apply direct pressure with a sterile pad or clean, dry cloth until the bleeding subsides. Do not remove the first pad if it becomes soaked, place a second one over it. If possible, elevate the area.
- All animal bites that break the skin carry the risk of tetanus. Visit a doctor for an antitetanus booster unless your immunization is up to date.
- Seek immediate medical attention for all human bites. If you have not had an antitetanus shot within the last five years, get one after any injury in which the skin is broken. It is a good idea to have a booster every 10 years.

TETANUS AND RABIES

Tetanus is caused by toxins that live in soil and in the intestines of humans and animals and act on the nerves controlling muscle activity. Symptoms usually appear five to 10 days after infection and include fever, headache, and muscle stiffness in the jaw (lockjaw), arms, neck and back. Painful muscle spasms may affect the throat or chest wall, leading to breathing difficulties. If you suspect tetanus, seek medical assistance without delay.

Rabies, a potentially fatal infection of the nervous system, is transmitted in saliva from the bite of a rabid animal. Early symptoms are flu-like, progressing to facial paralysis, thirst, throat spasms, disorientation and coma. If treated early, the chance of recovery is good. Rabies is rare in developed countries, but any bite should be followed by a visit to the doctor for a vaccination.

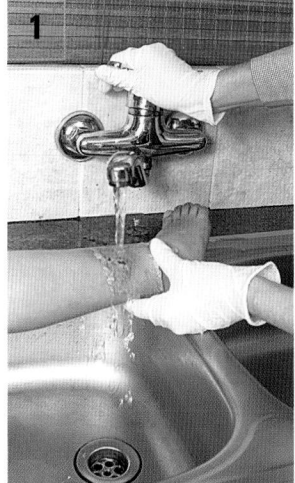 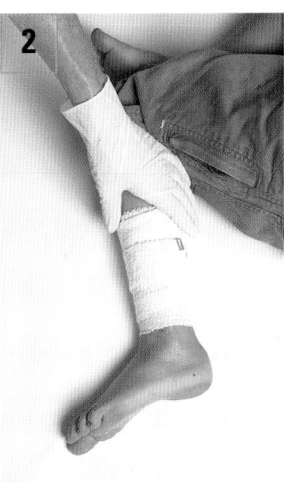

1. *Run the bite wound under the tap for three to five minutes to wash it.*
2. *Cover the wound with an antiseptic ointment and a clean dressing.*

INSECT BITES AND STINGS

Flying insects:

- A sting from a flying insect usually causes a painful red swelling which gets better within 24 hours. The only danger is if there are multiple stings and a large amount of venom is injected, which can cause toxic reactions such as fever, vomiting, and kidney malfunction. Anyone who is allergic will have a more severe reaction

Crawling insects:

- The bite of the brown spider causes local pain, swelling and a slow-healing, blister-like sore. Black widow, button and funnel web spiders inject venom which attacks the nervous system, causing muscle paralysis and breathing difficulties
- Most scorpion stings cause severe local pain and sensitivity to touch, heat and cold, but some can cause muscle pains or spasms, a general sense of weakness, coma and convulsions

There are more insects and spiders on earth than just about any other life form and, while most are harmless, or at best an irritation, there are some that are harmful, being able to deliver a bite or sting that is painful or potentially deadly. If bitten or stung by an insect, try to capture or kill it (if this can be done safely), so that it can be identified.

CAUSES

Flying insects sting anything or anyone who disturbs them or their nests or hives. The risk is generally highest in summer, particularly if you are active outdoors. Crawling insects sting when disturbed, often by lifting a rock or piece of wood. Even seemingly 'dead' insects can sting, so warn children not to pick them up.

Flying insects:

- Bees (honeybee, bumblebee).
- Wasps, hornets and yellow jackets.

Crawling insects:

- Spiders (black widow, brown recluse/violin spider, funnel web, button), scorpions.
- Ticks, fleas, ants and bedbugs.

PREVENTION

- Don't provoke the animals and avoid rapid, jerky movements around hives or nests.
- Use appropriate insect repellents on all exposed skin and/or protective clothing.
- Be vigilant when eating outdoors, especially with colas or sweetened beverages, which attract bees.

EMERGENCY DRUGS

If anyone in the family is known to be allergic to insect bites or stings, your doctor may advise you to keep a pre-packed adrenaline pen or syringe in your first aid kit. Given into the thigh muscle, this may be life-saving in the event of a severe allergic or anaphylactic reaction, but it must be given correctly. Follow your doctor's advice, and read the package instructions carefully before use.

KNOW YOUR INSECTS

Bees

A honeybee's stinger usually remains in the skin. Do not try to remove it using your fingers, as you will probably squeeze the poison sac and inject more venom. Instead, scrape the blunt edge of a knife-blade or a credit card across the stinger to remove it without injecting more venom. An alternative is to use a pair of fine tweezers, grasp the stinger as close as possible to the skin and not by the poison sac.

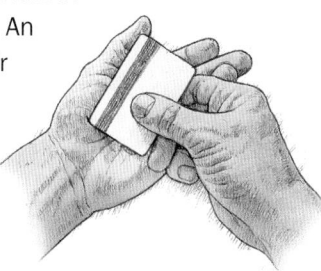

Ticks

These parasites attach themselves to a person's skin and suck their blood. Ticks can be as tiny as a pinhead or a large as a fingernail. They live in areas of dense forest, in shrub and in tall grass, and can adhere to any part of your body, from your feet to your arms and head.

The unpleasant symptoms of tick-bite fever include a red rash around the area of the bite, a feeling of tiredness, raging headache and flu-like fever. Make an appointment to see your doctor if you suspect that you may have contracted tickbite fever.

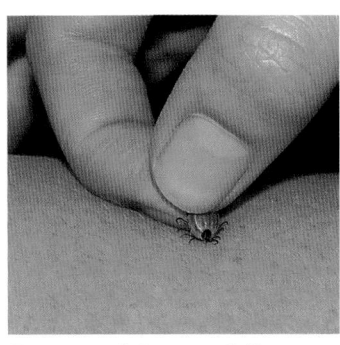

Remove ticks carefully to prevent mouth parts remaining embedded in the skin.

Some ticks can cause Lyme disease, an infection that, if untreated, results in muscle and joint pain and can affect the heart and nervous system.

The best way to prevent a tick bite is to cover as much of the body as you can when walking in long grass or the bush. Wear closed shoes or boots with long socks, and tuck long pants into your socks. Light-coloured clothing makes it easier to spot a tick. When you return home, shake out your clothing before putting it into the wash, checking that no ticks fall to the floor. Thoroughly check your body, paying attention to the scalp, groin, armpits and the back of knees. Because ticks are sometimes hidden by swelling around the bite, it is important to check any lumps carefully.

TREATMENT

Complications from insect bites and stings include reaction to the toxic venom, infection at the site of the bite, and shock. Allergic reactions to insect bites or stings usually occur within minutes. Severe allergic reactions (known as **anaphylaxis**, *see* p42), can cause breathing difficulties and can be rapidly fatal if untreated.

- Check ABC (*see* pp22–3). Begin **rescue breathing** (*see* p26) or **chest compressions** (*see* pp22–37) if necessary. Call for emergency assistance.
- If the casualty has a severe reaction or has been stung inside the mouth or throat, call immediately for medical assistance.
- Keep the casualty calm and still, as anxiety and movement will speed the distribution of the venom through the body. If appropriate, treat for **shock** (*see* p40). Remain with the casualty until medical help arrives.
- Remove watches, rings and constricting items because the affected area may swell.
- If the pain is severe or does not subside within a few hours, get the casualty to a doctor. In the interim, keep the casualty immobile to reduce the spread of the poison. If breathing becomes compromised, begin rescue breathing.
- If emergency assistance is not required, wash the bite or sting site with soap and water and cover it with a clean, cold compress, ice pack, or a clean, moist dressing to reduce swelling and discomfort.
- Take a mild analgesic to relieve the pain.
- Over the next 24–48 hours, observe the site for signs of infection (such as redness, swelling, ulceration or increasing pain).

SPIDERS, SCORPIONS AND SNAKES

SPIDERS

Most spiders bite if they are disturbed, so avoid breaking or brushing against webs, and take care when working in the garden, as spiders often live under rocks and in any handy crevice. Many bites occur at night, when someone rolls onto a nocturnal invader in their sleep. Spider venom is neurotoxic (it affects the central nervous system). In severe cases, bites can cause breathing problems and an irregular heartbeat, leading to loss of consciousness and death.

SCORPIONS AND CENTIPEDES

Although scorpions and centipedes can deliver a painful sting, few are lethal, unless the casualty is a child. As with spiders, scorpions attack if they are disturbed in their natural habitat, so be careful when lifting stones or pieces of wood. Scorpions are nocturnal and spend the daylight hours under rocks, logs and in places that provide shade and protection. If you are camping in areas where scorpions are found, check your boots before putting them on in the morning!

SNAKES

Some 300 of the 2000-plus species of snake are dangerous to man. Depending on the species, snake venom is neurotoxic, haemotoxic, or cytotoxic. Regard all snake bites as a medical emergency, and get the casualty to an emergency room as quickly as possible, as the administration of the right anti-venom can save a life. Because of their small body size, children are at higher risk for complications or death. Most people know when they have been bitten but, in the event that someone is found unconscious, symptoms to look out are puncture marks in the skin made by the fangs, swelling or skin discoloration at the site of the bite, difficulty in breathing and a rapid pulse. A conscious casualty may experience numbness and a general sense of weakness, blurred vision, fever, nausea, dizziness, fainting, and loss of muscle coordination, along with excessive sweating, convulsions and increased thirst.

TREATMENT

- Obtain medical help immediately. Meanwhile, keep the casualty calm and restrict movement, as exertion will cause the venom to circulate faster through the body. Keep the affected area below heart level to reduce the flow of venom.
- Monitor the casualty's vital signs (pulse, breathing, and blood pressure). If there are signs of shock lay the casualty flat, raise the feet about 30cm (12in), and cover him with a blanket.
- If a bite is on the hand or arm, remove rings, watches etc., as the limb may swell.
- Apply a large, overlapping pressure bandage to the bite site and up the full length of the limb. Move the limb as little as possible, and use a splint to keep it still.
- Venom can cause partial blindness, so if any enters the eyes, rinse them immediately with water. Wipe away venom near the eyes and prevent the casualty from rubbing the eyes, even though they will want to.
- Don't remove venom on unbroken skin as it can be analyzed to identify the snake, if identification is not possible by other means.

Wrap a bandage from the bite up to the armpit.

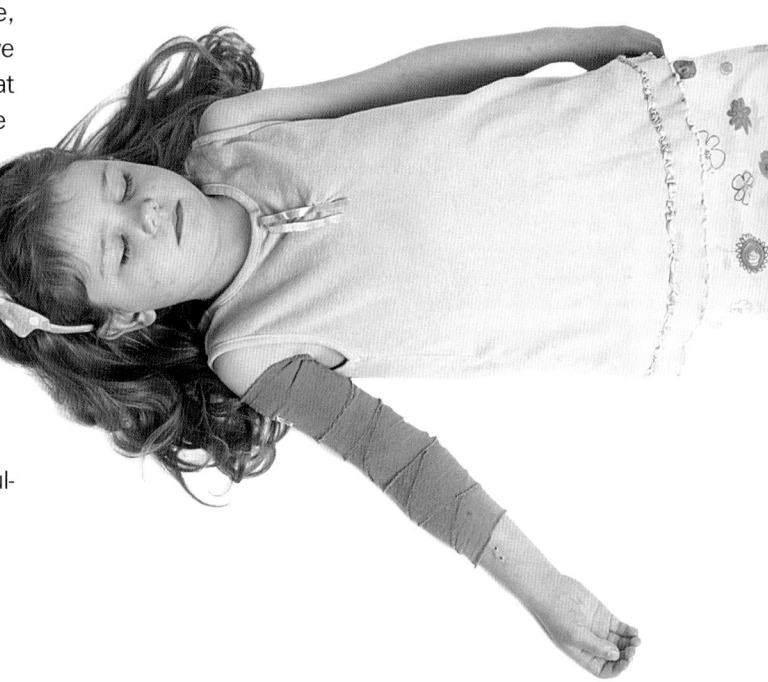

MARINE CREATURES

Several animals and organisms living in the sea are capable of delivering a variety of bites and stings. Encounters with coral, sea urchins, cone shells and a variety of molluscs can result in scratches and lacerations. And the nematocysts that are found on the tentacles of jellyfish and on sea anemones are capable of delivering nasty injuries.

The bigger fish such as barracudas, eels, rays and sharks can give a severe bite, while the venomous spines of stonefish and scorpion fish can inflict a painful wound. Electric eels are capable of delivering severe electrical shocks. Even one's dinner can fight back, and there are probably few anglers who have never been on the receiving end of a sharp bite from a fish that looked dead!

The most common reason for a bite or sting is that the marine creature has been disturbed in its natural habitat. Children who are busy exploring rock pools, and snorkellers leisurely inspecting a coast line or reef are most at risk, but swimmers and fishermen can also fall victim if they happen to have an unexpected encounter. As with all wildlife, the best remedy is to give marine creatures a wide berth and respect their habitat and environment.

TREATMENT

- If there is a trained life guard on the beach – call him or her to come and help you.
- Wear gloves when removing stingers to avoid getting stung yourself.
- Keep the casualty quiet and still to reduce the movement of toxins around the body.
- Pour vinegar or dilute acetic acid (5–10%) over the site to deactivate the stinging cells.
- Once the stingers are deactivated, remove tentacles by lifting them off with a stick – wiping them off can cause further stinging.
- Rinse the affected area with sea water to wash away any nematocysts that have remained on the skin.
- A sunburn preparation containing lidocaine or benzocaine will act as a mild anaesthetic to reduce the pain.
- Use cold compresses (ice blocks) to reduce inflammation, itching and redness.
- If the casualty develops persistent muscle spasms, seek medical attention.
- Seek medical attention if vesicles (blisters) form, as they can result in infection.

SYMPTOMS

- Localized pain, burning, swelling, redness
- Weakness, faintness, dizziness
- Difficulty in breathing or painful breathing
- Cramps and muscle weakness
- Fever and sweating
- Pain in the groin and armpits
- Nausea, vomiting or diarrhoea
- Runny nose, excessive tears
- Irregular pulse
- Paralysis

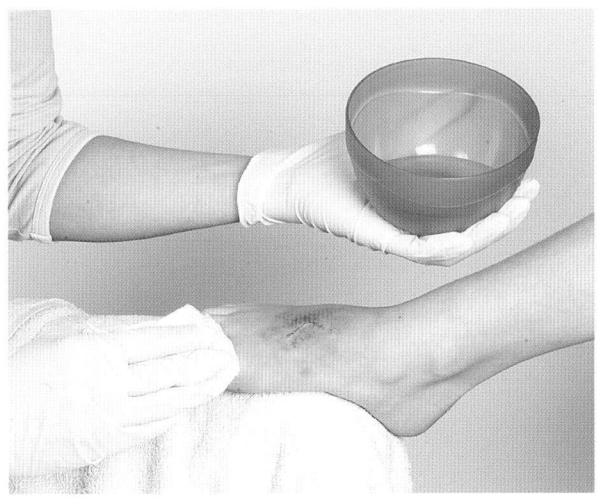

Wash a jellyfish sting with vinegar to restrict the poison from being fired from the tentacles.

Aches and pains

Although pain is an experience most people would choose to avoid, it does serve an important function, warning us that all is not well in some area or system of the body. Pain occurs when specialized nerve endings, known as pain fibres, which are distributed widely throughout the body, are irritated, damaged, or come under pressure. Pain is an early warning sign of illness or injury, telling us that we need to pay attention to the cause, as well as taking a painkiller for relief.

SYMPTOMS

- Pain associated with acute injury will resolve as the injury recovers. Large bruises or blood clots under the skin may be tender for several days.
- An irritation or obstruction of the digestive tract causes a cramping sensation which comes and goes. Infants and small children are not able to describe this, but it should be suspected if a child cries lustily, drawing up their legs periodically, with quiet intervals in between.
- Sudden sharp pain in the knees, hips or lower back, brought on by physical exertion, or lifting heavy objects, may be due to complications of osteo-arthritis, particularly in older people.
- Lower back pain that radiates down the back of a leg may be caused by nerve compression from a 'slipped' disc between the vertebrae.
- Severe pain which affects the joints of the foot, particularly at night, may be due to gout. Typically, the affected joint is swollen, and the skin is red and very tender to touch.

CAUSES

- Injury is by far the most common cause of aches and pains, which may come on abruptly after a specific injury, or increase over time through repetitive injury to bones, joints, ligaments and tendons as a result of sport or physical exertion.
- Pain is frequently a symptom of infection, obstruction, chemical irritation or stretching of the digestive, respiratory, urinary or genital tracts.
- The wear and tear of degenerative bone disease, which occurs with advancing age, may cause bones in the weight-bearing parts of the skeleton (hips, knees and lower back) to slip out of alignment with one another, or press on nerves, causing pain associated with movement, as well as stiffness on getting up in the morning.
- Any enlarging mass inside a confined space, for example a tumour, may cause varying degrees of pain, depending on the rate of growth, and the room available for expansion. Therefore, a tumour inside the skull will often cause severe headache, while a tumour of similar size inside the abdomen may cause no discomfort at all.
- Infection in any part of the body may become localized to form an abscess, which can cause persistent excruciating pain, disrupt sleep, and may be associated with fever. Superficial abscesses are red, tender swellings, but some may be deep-seated and difficult to spot.
- Localized head pain may be caused by a **headache or migraine** (*see* p98).
- Adolescents can experience 'growing pains' during the growth spurts that take place during puberty.

TREATMENT

- Treatment of aches and pains should consist of symptomatic pain relief, while ensuring that the underlying cause is identified and dealt with.
- For pain relief, always use the mildest possible analgesic. Over-the-counter painkillers such as paracetamol/acetaminophen and aspirin are generally safe, and should always be used as a first option. Cramping pain caused by disorders of the gut or urinary tract may require medication which only a doctor can prescribe. Bone or joint pain often responds best to anti-inflammatory medication, such as ibuprofen, which should be taken in consultation with a doctor due to the risk of stomach irritation and other potential side-effects.
- The severe pain of an abscess will only be relieved by surgical drainage of the pus.
- Toothache usually implies tooth decay or infection and should be investigated by a dentist as soon as possible.
- Acute gout can be prevented by avoiding certain foods and taking medication that blocks the production of uric acid. See your doctor about a long-term treatment plan.

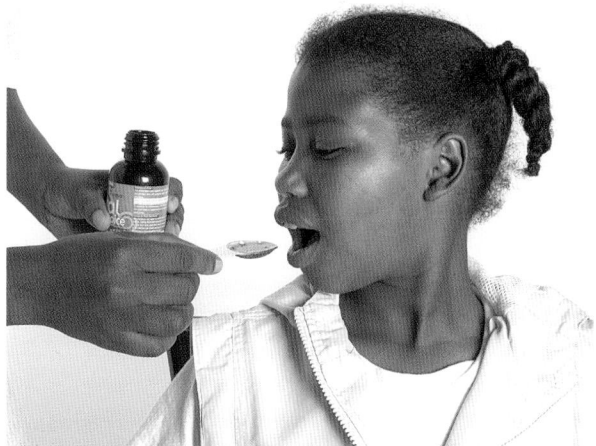

Syrup-based painkiller is best for young children and those who cannot swallow tablets.

PREVENTION

Pain is a normal physiological response to both illness and injury, and an important warning symptom which should be heeded in good time. In most instances, pain can't be prevented, but you can ensure that the cause of the pain is diagnosed and treated appropriately before a mild condition develops into a serious one.

By all means, treat a single episode of pain with a painkiller, but do not hesitate to see a doctor if pain persists, recurs, or does not respond to over-the-counter drugs.

SEEK MEDICAL HELP IF:

- there is pain in any part of the body for 24 hours or more, or pain that recurs on a regular basis.
- painkillers have to be taken with increasing frequency, or in increasing doses.
- there are abdominal cramps associated with vomiting or changes in bowel habits.
- there is a cramping pain in either side, particularly if there is blood in the urine.
- there is a painful swelling.
- a lower back pain begins to radiate down the back of the leg.

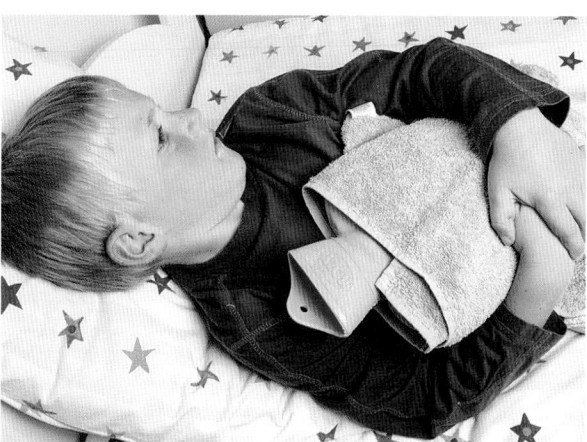

A hot-water bottle and bedrest are good solutions to easing a nagging pain.

Heat exhaustion and heatstroke

Heat exhaustion and heatstroke usually result from a combination of hot environmental conditions and physical exertion. In hot weather we sweat, resulting in a loss of fluid and salts, which causes the body to become dehydrated, resulting in heat exhaustion. If preventative steps are not taken, blood pressure can drop and the pulse rate can slow, causing a casualty to faint. If there is continued exposure to heat, the body may not be able to cool itself by sweating. The result is a rapid rise in body temperature – a life-threatening condition known as heatstroke. Both heat exhaustion and heatstroke can be avoided by taking a few precautions. Children, the obese and the elderly are most at risk, but even an athlete in peak condition can succumb if warning signs are ignored.

SYMPTOMS

Although heatstroke may be preceded by a headache, dizziness and fatigue, it often comes on quickly, bringing fever, a high temperature (above 40°C/104°F), and rapid pulse rate (over 160 beats per minute). Untreated, heatstroke can result in coma, brain damage and, in extreme cases, death due to kidney failure. Early signs are:

- Excessive sweating
- Fatigue
- Muscle cramps
- Dizziness and faintness
- Headache
- Nausea and vomiting

If exposure to heat continues, the following may develop:

- Increase in body temperature
- Increased pulse rate and rapid, shallow breathing
- Hot, dry and red skin
- Feelings of anxiety and confusion
- Weakness, light-headedness
- Irrational behaviour
- Seizures

CAUSES

- Continued exposure to very hot weather (external temperatures above 35°C/95°F), particularly when coupled with high humidity (averaging 50 per cent or more).
- Performing physical labour or exercising excessively in hot weather.
- Engaging in endurance or competitive sport, particularly when physically unfit.
- Wearing too much clothing in hot weather.

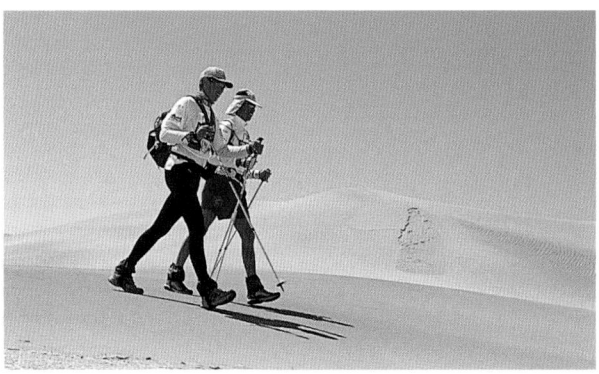

Remember to drink plenty of fluids in hot weather.

TREATMENT

HEAT EXHAUSTION

The condition will usually resolve itself with rest in a cool place and the intake of fluids (non-alcoholic, non-carbonated beverages). Avoid drinks containing caffeine. Encourage the casualty to drink small quantities every hour or so until they feel recovered. Removing unnecessary clothing and sponging the body with tepid water will lower the temperature.

Summon medical assistance immediately if the casualty's condition does not improve, deteriorates or their level of alertness changes (they become confused, or unconscious or suffer from seizures).

TREATMENT FOR HEATSTROKE

While waiting for help to arrive:

- Lie the casualty down in a cool area, feet raised about 30cm (12in).
- Apply wet cloths to the skin, soak in tepid water, or apply cold compresses to the neck, armpits and groin. Use an electic fan, or a magazine or board, to create a flow of cool air around the casualty.
- If the casualty is alert, provide cool non-alcoholic, non-carbonated drinks or administer salt solution (*see* p108) every 15 minutes. If you don't have either, plain cool water will do.
- Administer first aid for **shock** (*see* p40).
- If **seizures** (*see* p44) occur, protect the casualty from injury, and administer first aid.
- If the casualty is **unconscious** (*see* p22–37), give appropriate first aid.
- Be aware of complications if the casualty has medical problems such as high blood pressure.

CAUTION

Heatstroke is a medical emergency and requires hospitalization. **Call for assistance without delay**.

X DO NOT

- use an alcohol rub to cool the casualty.
- underestimate heatstroke or heat exhaustion as they can be serious, particularly in children, the elderly or injured.
- provide medication, such as aspirin, that is used to treat fever.
- provide anything at all by mouth if the casualty is vomiting or unconscious.
- permit someone suffering from heatstroke to resume physical activity as soon as they feel better.

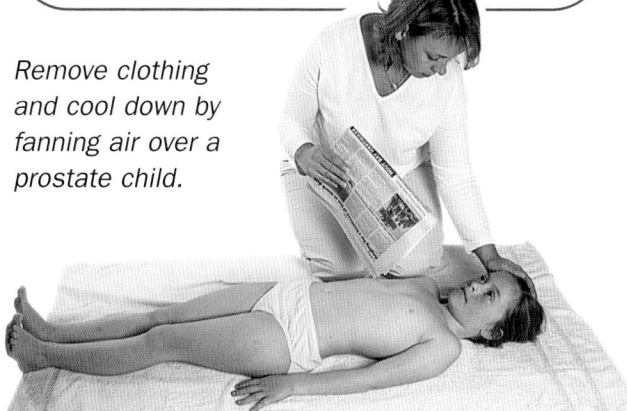

Remove clothing and cool down by fanning air over a prostate child.

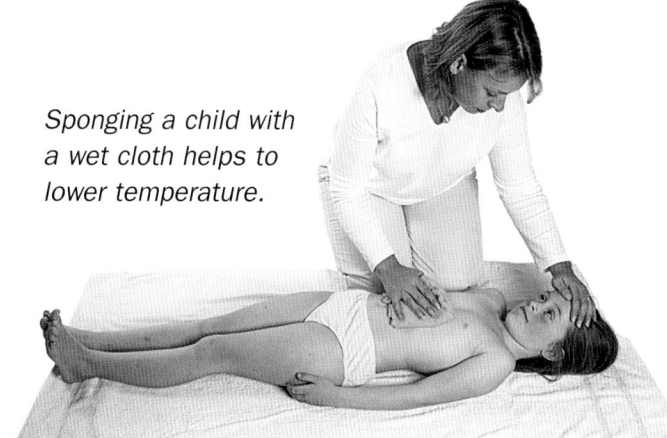

Sponging a child with a wet cloth helps to lower temperature.

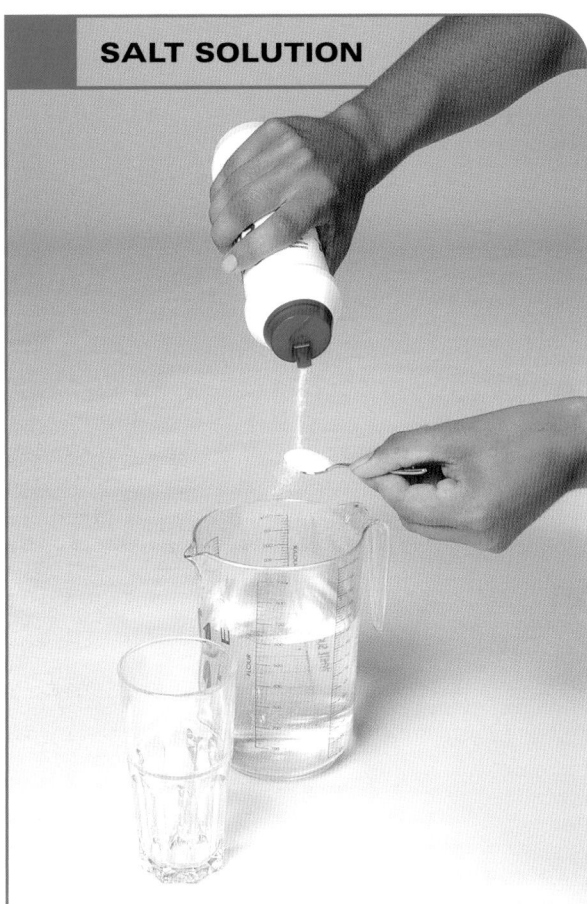

SALT SOLUTION

Mix one teaspoon of salt to one litre/two pints of water and give the casualty about half a cup (125ml) every 15 minutes. If you don't have cool drinks or salt available, plain cool water is better than nothing.

Place a child suffering from heat exhaustion in the shade and give her a drink of water.

PREVENTION

- Increase both salt and fluid intake when exercising in hot weather.
- Rather drink too many fluids than too few, but beware of overhydration.
- Avoid strenuous outdoor activity in the heat of the day. If you work or play sport in a hot and humid environment, take regular rest periods in cooler areas, either indoors or in the shade.
- Wear light, loose clothing and a hat with a broad brim. This applies particularly to children playing outdoors in very hot weather.
- If you are elderly, obese or on medication that impairs your body's heat regulation mechanism, avoid overheating.
- Tourists are often at risk of heat exhaustion. If you are travelling to the tropics, allow yourself time to acclimatize before you exert yourself.

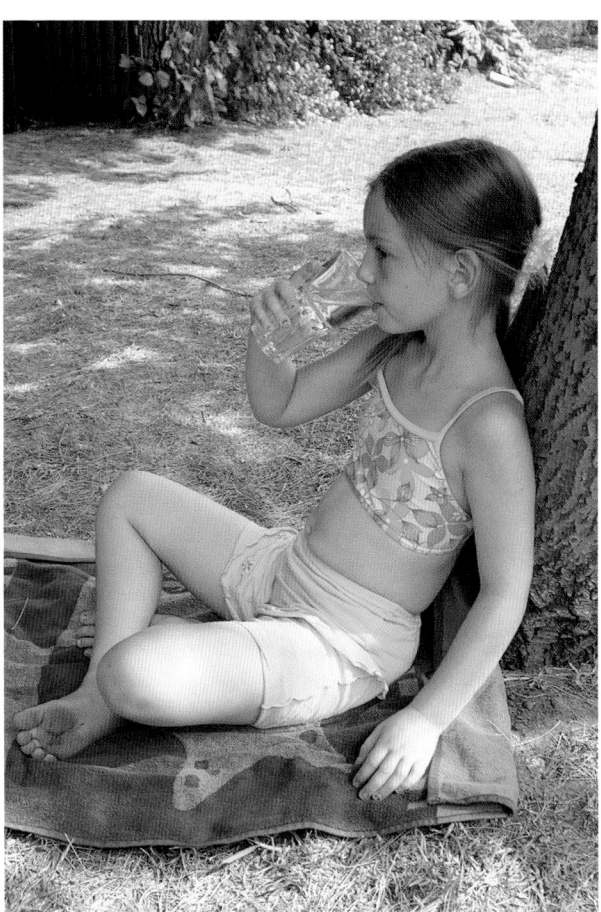

Hypothermia

Hypothermia occurs when the body loses more heat than it can generate, usually by being exposed to cold for an extended period. It is characterized by a low body temperature, below 35°C (95°F). The

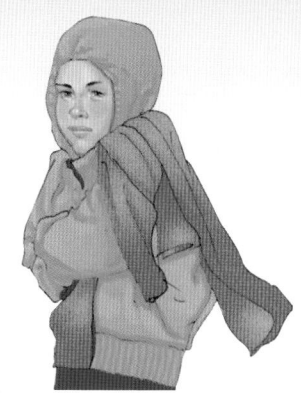

symptoms of hypothermia develop relatively slowly, affecting the person's mental and physical state, leading to apathy, lethargy and drowsiness. This means the casualty might not detect hypothermia and may fail to take preventative measures either soon enough, or to the necessary degree.

Generally, people with a chronic illness, such as a heart or circulation problem, the very old or very young, and those who are tired, malnourished, or under the influence of drugs or alcohol are at risk of hypothermia when subjected to conditions which could bring it about.

SYMPTOMS

- Pale and cold skin
- Apathy, lethargy and drowsiness
- Weakness
- Slurred speech
- Confusion
- Shock
- Slowed breathing or heart rate
- Coma
- Cardiac arrest
- The casualty might shiver uncontrollably but shivering can stop when the body temperature is extremely low

CAUSES
Factors that contribute to hypothermia include the following:
- Cold weather, particularly when accompanied by wind, which causes a chill factor that lowers the body temperature further than it would drop in similar calm conditions.
- Immersion in cold water.
- Exposure to excessive cold by being outside without sufficient protective clothing.
- Continuing to wear wet clothing for an extended period of time in cold, wet and/or windy conditions.

 CAUTION

Hypothermia needs prompt treatment as it can be fatal. The most extreme symptoms – cardiac arrest, shock and coma – can set in if initial first aid measures are ineffective or are not carried out promptly.

- Heavy exertion outdoors in cold weather.
- Continual exposure to cold conditions while under the influence of certain medications or alcohol.
- Poor circulation resulting from excessively tight clothing or from lying in one position for too long. Fatigue, alcohol consumption, certain medications and smoking can all impede circulation.
- Insufficient consumption of suitable hot foods and liquids to 'fuel' the body in very cold weather.

TREATMENT

- Get the casualty into a warm environment as quickly as possible and summon medical assistance.
- Remove wet clothing. If garments are dry, loosen tight cuffs and collars – not forgetting the legs and the ankle area.
- Place the casualty on a blanket or coat to insulate against a cold floor and cover with blankets. Much body heat is lost via the top of the head, which is richly supplied with blood, so keep the head and neck region well covered.
- Apply warm compresses to the neck, chest and groin area, and keep the head warm.
- If the casualty is conscious, alert and able to swallow without choking, give warm non-alcoholic sweetened fluids to speed up the warming process.

- If it is very cold and you cannot get the casualty to a warm place, at least get them out of the wind and into a relatively sheltered area. Cover them warmly and be sure to protect them from the cold ground.
- Remain with the casualty until help arrives.

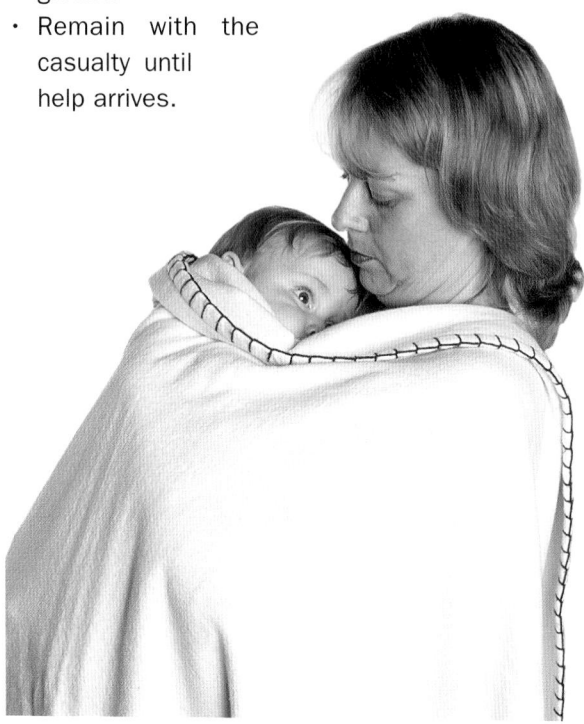

Use your own body heat and a blanket to rewarm a cold infant.

People suffering from hypothermia should not only be warmed from the outside, serve a warm drink to warm them inside.

 DO NOT

- assume that a person found motionless in the cold is dead. Get the inert body to shelter, begin **rescue breathing** (*see* p26) and/or **chest compressions** (*see* pp22–37) if necessary, and provide the above-mentioned first aid measures.
- try to warm the casualty by applying direct heat such as hot water, a heating pad or a heat lamp. If the casualty's senses are so dulled that they do not react, your actions could result in burns.
- give the casualty alcohol to drink, even after recovery.

STAGES OF HYPOTHERMIA

MILD
Core temperature 35ºC–32ºC
(95ºF–92ºF)

- Complains of severe cold
- Poor judgement, confusion, irritability
- Slurred speech, stumbling
- Uncontrollable shivering
- Cold, blue hands and feet
- Stiff muscles
- High urine production leading to dehydration

MODERATE
Core temperature 32ºC–28ºC
(90ºF–82.4ºF)

- Decreased level of consciousness
- Shivering may stop
- Muscles are stiff and rigid
- Irregular heartbeat

SEVERE
Temperature below 28ºC
(82.2ºF)–Core temperature

- Deeply unconscious
- Slow breathing
- Slow, irregular heartbeat
- Heart may stop

is much easier to spot a car than a person. If you decide to abandon your vehicle, leave a prominently displayed message giving your departure time, direction of travel, mobile phone number and any other information that might aid those looking for you.

- Take care that babies and small children are adequately insulated and protected from the cold, especially at night. If there is any doubt, rather let them sleep with you.
- While hiking, make a mental note of landmarks and potential shelters along the way.

PREVENTION

- Wear head gear to keep your head warm and slow the loss of heat from the top of the head.
- Wear mittens rather than gloves, and gloves rather than nothing.
- Wear suitable clothing and protect exposed, sensitive areas. Clothing should be wind-proof and water-resistant, and preferably, multilayered.
- Avoid wet or constricting clothing – beware of tight cuffs, leggings, or footwear that impede circulation to the extremities (often at greater risk anyway).
- Wear two pairs of socks (cotton next to skin, wool next to footwear) and water-resistant footwear that provides protection at least to the ankles. Warm and dry feet in cold conditions are important.
- Beware of going out in extremely cold conditions, and wear suitable gear when diving, surfing or taking part in other water-related activities.
- If you are on medication, check with your doctor, as some medicines might interfere with your blood circulation and/or blood pressure.
- If your vehicle breaks down or gets stuck in unfamiliar terrain, stay with it. In adverse conditions, it

WAYS OF PRODUCING HEAT

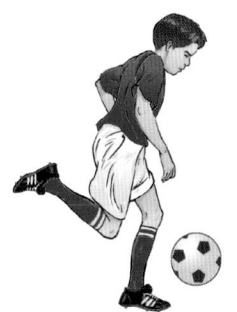

Physical activity

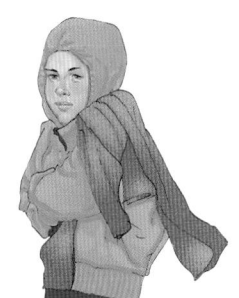

Warm clothing

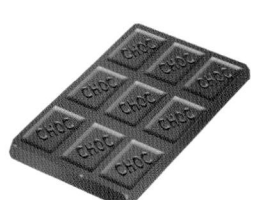

High-energy food

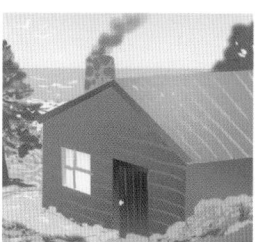

Heated shelter

Frostbite

Frostbite is the damage extreme cold can do to the skin and underlying tissues. It usually occurs on the extremities (face, nose, ears, hands, fingers and feet), which tend to be more exposed. As with many conditions, the duration and extent of exposure determine the extent of the damage. The pressure of wind chill, together with low temperatures, increases the risk of frostbite as well as **hypothermia** (*see* p115).

SYMPTOMS

- A sensation of 'pins and needles' is the first symptom.
- Numbness, throbbing or aching may follow, after which sensation (feeling) is lost completely as the affected part starts to feel like a 'block of wood' and the skin becomes hard, pale and cold.
- As the tissue affected by early frostbite thaws it becomes red and painful.
- In extreme cases, the skin will become numb and turn white as the tissue freezes. This may be accompanied by blisters and gangrene (blackened dead tissue). Bone, tendons, muscles and nerves might also be damaged.

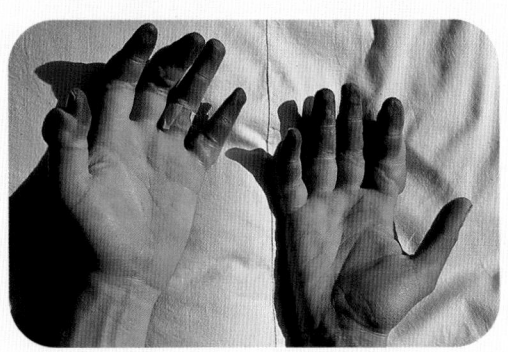

CAUSES

Anyone who is exposed to freezing cold for a prolonged period can get frostbite. Inadequate clothing and insufficient protection for the head, hands and feet exacerbate the problem; as do external factors like wind chill.

With adequate shelter and protection, most people can survive just about any weather condition, but the risk is increased by certain factors, such as taking beta-blockers (which decrease the flow of blood to the skin), smoking, being inebriated, and chronic conditions like diabetes and low blood pressure.

PREVENTION

- When venturing outdoors in icy weather, wear wind- and waterproof clothing with multi-layered upper-body protection; mittens or gloves; and a hood, scarf or woollen cap (you lose most body heat via the top of your head). Ensure cuffs are snug but not so tight they constrict the flow of blood to your hands.
- Choose well-fitting, water-resistant footwear and wear two pairs of socks: cotton next to your skin, then wool.
- If caught outdoors in very cold weather or snow, find shelter or increase physical activity to maintain body warmth.
- Be aware of factors that affect the blood vessels, such as smoking, alcohol, medication, and conditions such as low blood pressure or diabetes.
- If bad weather threatens when you are hiking, make a note of potential shelter along the route; if a storm strikes, you will know where to find refuge.

TREATMENT

- Get the casualty into warm surroundings and protect them from further cold. Remove wet or constricting clothing and jewellery, substituting it for something warm and loose. Blankets are ideal if no warm, dry clothing is available.
- Look for signs of **hypothermia** (*see* p115) and treat accordingly .
- Wrap the affected parts in sterile dressings (wrap toes and fingers individually to keep them separated) and get the casualty to a medical facility for further care.
- When medical care is not immediately available, immerse the affected areas in warm, not hot, water (about 40–42°C/104–108°F), or repeatedly apply warm cloths to the frostbitten area for about 30 minutes.
- When immersing the frostbitten area, circulate the water with your hand as this will aid the warming process. The casualty may experience severe burning pain and swelling, and the affected part may change colour during warming. Warming is complete when the skin is soft and sensation has returned to the affected area.
- Provide warm, sweetened drinks.
- If there is a chance that frostbitten parts may freeze again and you are far from medical help or warm shelter, then delay first aid procedures until the chance of refreezing has been eliminated. Tissue damage can be exacerbated if frostbite thaws and then refreezes, whereas if it is kept in a steady state and thawed once only, the damage may be lessened.
- Always have frostbite checked by a doctor, even if you have made a complete recovery. Seek medical assistance if recovery is not complete or new symptoms develop. (These include fever, malaise, discolouration of the frostbitten area and seeping or oozing of fluids from the area.)

X DO NOT

- disturb blisters on frostbitten skin.
- immerse a frostbitten area in hot water as the scalding would increase the risk of tissue damage (use warm water only).
- rub or massage a frostbitten area.
- smoke or consume alcohol during recovery, as this can interfere with blood circulation and slow the recovery process.
- thaw a frostbitten area if it cannot be kept thawed, as refreezing may make tissue damage even worse.
- use direct dry heat (from sources such as hair dryers or heating pads) to thaw the frostbitten areas, as you may apply excessive heat, burning the skin and causing more damage.

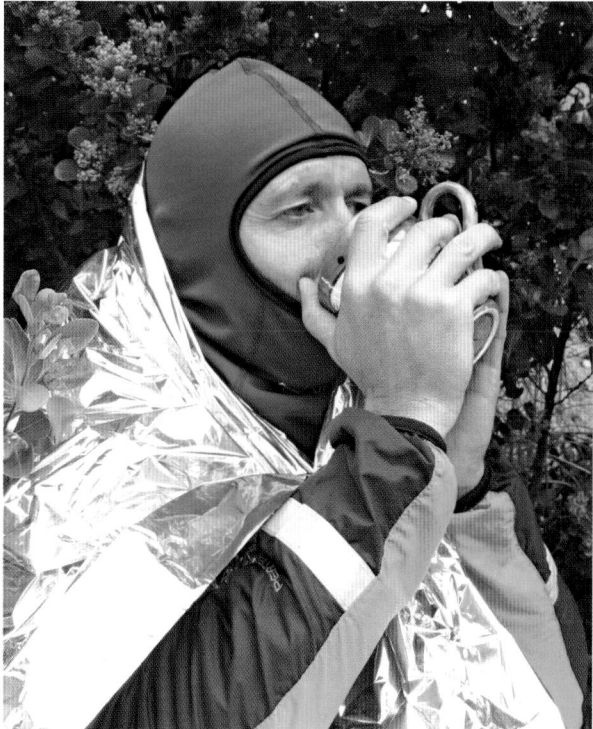

Rewarm a frozen person with a survival blanket and a warm beverage.

Electrical shock

An electrical shock occurs when the body, or part of it, becomes a conduit for electricity from a strong source to an area of lower electrical energy. The extent of the injury is determined by the size and duration of the shock, the level of conductivity between the body and whatever it is touching, and the route the current took as it travelled through the body. Depending on its severity, an electric shock can cause damage to nerves, muscles and other tissues, as well as thermal burns ranging from comparatively minor to very serious. Even if an electrical burn looks slight, the shock could have resulted in internal damage to the heart, muscles, or brain, which can result in cardiac arrest.

SYMPTOMS

- Sudden, unexplained loss of consciousness, particularly when the shock was not witnessed by another person
- Skin burns
- Muscular pain
- Numbness, tingling
- Muscle contraction with residual pain, for a while at least
- Headache
- Weakness
- Hearing impairment
- Irregular pulse
- Seizures
- Respiratory failure
- Unconsciousness
- Cardiac arrest

CAUSES

- Accidental contact with exposed wiring or unearthed parts of electrical appliances
- Incorrect connection of appliance plugs or wiring
- Children chewing on electrical cords, or poking metal objects into an electrical outlet, such as a plug socket
- Lightning strikes
- Laying electrical cords under rugs, resulting in damage to the insulation
- Accidentally cutting underground power cables while doing maintenance work
- Exposure to unearthed power tools or machinery
- Flashing (electric arcs) from high-voltage power lines

TREATMENT

- Once the casualty is free from the source of electricity, check their ABC (*see* pp22–3). If any funcations have ceased or seem dangerously slow or shallow, initiate **resuscitation** (*see* pp22–37).
- If the casualty has a burn, remove any clothing that comes off easily, cool the injury in running water until the pain subsides and administer first aid for **burns** (*see* p52).
- If the casualty is showing signs of **shock** (*see* p40), lie them down with the head slightly lower than the body and the legs elevated, and cover them with a blanket.
- If the shock has caused the casualty to fall (off a

ladder, for instance), there could be internal injuries. If you suspect a spinal injury, avoid moving the casualty's head or neck. Administer appropriate first aid for wounds or **fractures** (*see* p68).
- Stay with the casualty until professional medical help arrives.

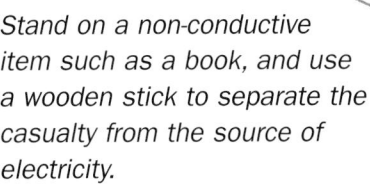

Stand on a non-conductive item such as a book, and use a wooden stick to separate the casualty from the source of electricity.

Or use a towel or rope to pull the person out of harm's way.

✗ DO NOT

- touch the casualty with your bare hands while the person is still in contact with the source of electricity.
- get within 6m (20ft) of someone who is being electrocuted by high-voltage electrical current until the power is turned off.
- move a casualty unless he or she is in any immediate danger.

PREVENTION

- Always treat electricity with respect and teach your children about the dangers of electricity.
  - Keep electrical appliances and cords out of children's reach and make sure they never play with any cord – even a piece you have discarded. Next time it might be attached to a wall socket.
- Use child safety plugs in all outlets.
- Never touch electrical appliances while touching taps (faucets) or water pipes.
- Follow the manufacturer's safety instructions when using electrical appliances or tools. Avoid using electrical appliances while wet, or when standing in a wet or damp patch – for instance in the early morning when dew is on the ground.
- If working up a ladder and using a power tool, choose a wooden rather than an alumimium ladder. Wood is a poor conductor of electricity.
- If you do not know how to wire an electric plug, then don't! Get a handyman or electrician do it.
- Always wear rubber-soled footwear when operating power tools.

SWITCHING OFF ELECTRIC CURRENT

Before you deal with the casualty, **switch off the electric current**. Use a piece of wood (broomstick or wooden spoon) to reach the switch. Do not put yourself at risk! If the current can't be turned off, use a dry non-conducting object such as a broom, chair, rug, or rubber doormat to push the casualty away from the source of the current. Don't use anything wet, damp or metallic. You may need to be rough – if the casualty has gripped the appliance, only a sharp tug or blow might break that grip and the contact. If possible, stand on something dry and non-conducting, such as a wooden plank, folded newspapers or a rubber or coir doormat while doing this.

Nausea and motion sickness

Nausea, the sensation of wanting to vomit, is a common symptom that usually does not require urgent medical attention. If, however, the condition is persistent, severe and/or prevents you keeping any food or drink down, then it may be a sign of something more serious. One of the main complications of vomiting is dehydration. The rate at which you become dehydrated depends on your size (infants can quickly become dehydrated as a result of persistent vomiting accompanied by diarrhoea), the frequency of the vomiting, and whether it is accompanied by diarrhoea.

SYMPTOMS

- An urge to vomit
- Actual vomiting
- A general feeling of unease or queasiness, particularly when at sea

CAUSES IN ADULTS
- Food allergies or food poisoning
- Viral infections
- Medications
- Seasickness or motion (car, air) sickness
- Morning sickness during pregnancy
- Accidental or deliberate ingestion of a drug or poison
- Alcoholism
- Bulimia
- Migraine headaches
- Chemotherapy

CAUSES IN INFANTS UP TO SIX MONTHS
- Overfeeding
- Being bounced excessively just after being fed
- Food allergies
- Milk intolerance
- Infection, often accompanied by fever/runny nose
- Intestinal obstruction, or a constriction in the outlet from the stomach, causing recurring attacks of vomiting and crying or screaming as if in great pain
- Poisoning
- Gastroenteritis
- Vomiting is a common sign of many infectious illnesses, including meningitis

TREATMENT
Whatever the cause of the vomiting, lost fluids should be restored as soon as possible; if not, dehydration can lead to other problems. Give water or diluted fruit juice, a sip at a time, as frequently as the patient can accept them without inducing more vomiting. The general rule is not too much food or liquid at once as the patient slowly works their way back to a normal diet.

TIP

For a home-made oral rehydration solution mix 1 teaspoon salt and 8 teaspoons sugar in 1 litre (2 pints) of cool, previously boiled water.

With infants and young children particularly, dehydration can develop very rapidly. If an infant is vomiting repeatedly, seek medical attention, and do not give the child more than a couple of teaspoons of water. Rather give a teaspoon every five minutes of half-strength formula or oral rehydration solution (keep some in the medicine cabinet – your doctor or pharmacist can advise you on a suitable product and dosages).

Since vomiting is almost always accompanied by some abdominal discomfort, generally you need be concerned only if the pain is severe.

DEHYDRATION

Suspect dehydration if a person complains of or exhibits any of the following:

· Being thirsty
· A dry mouth
· Eyes appear sunken
· Skin loses its normal elasticity
· Crying does not produce tears
· Infrequent or dark yellow urine

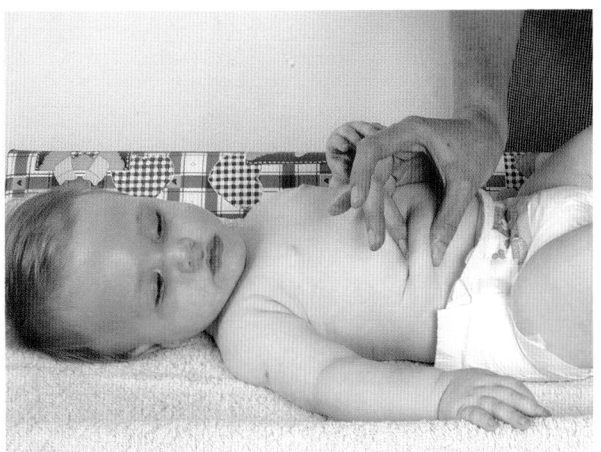

Gently pinch the side of the abdomen and if the raised skin does not return immediately to its normal position then suspect that dehydration has begun to set in.

MOTION SICKNESS

Some people are prone to motion sickness – either in a vehicle or at sea. Lying down will frequently help relieve the condition, as will the intake of fresh air, so open a window or get on deck. Looking ahead, at the horizon, rather than at the road or at moving water, also helps, as motion sickness occurs when the brain receives mixed messages from the eyes and the organs of balance in the inner ear. There are a number of proprietary medications aimed at preventing or reducing motion sickness. Ginger is often an effective remedy, so try ginger beer or biscuits (cookies) in small quantities.

PREVENTION

Attacks of nausea tend to occur suddenly and are very difficult to prevent, but you can reduce your susceptibility by taking the following steps:

Adults:
· Moderate your intake of rich foods and alcohol.
· Avoid eating food that appears 'off'.

Children:
· Follow normal feeding practices with infants, and avoid overfeeding.
· Guard against bacterial contamination of feeds, bottles, pacifiers and toys.

SEEK MEDICAL HELP IF:

● You suspect that a child has taken a drug or ingested a poisonous substance.

● The patient is vomiting and also displays any of the following symptoms:
· headache and/or stiff neck.
· an adult cannot retain any fluids for 12 hours or more.
· nausea persists for a prolonged period (apart from pregnant women, who may experience long periods of 'morning sickness').
· a young child becomes dehydrated and produces less urine than normal.
· a young child is lethargic, markedly irritable, and unable to retain fluids for eight hours or more, or vomiting recurs.

Home nursing and frail care

The cost of long-term hospitalization or frail care, coupled with the tedium and lack of intimacy and stimulation which characterize many institutions, may make home nursing an attractive option for ill, disabled or recovering elderly family members. Although the decision to nurse someone in your home is inevitably based on love and a deep sense of commitment, these sentiments alone are not enough. To succeed in practice, home nursing requires careful stocktaking of your own resources, planning, possibly some structural alterations, consultation with other family members and professionals and, of course, a budget. Here, we offer some general suggestions which should guide your decision as to whether home nursing is a viable option, and help you create the correct environment and other conditions necessary for successful home care.

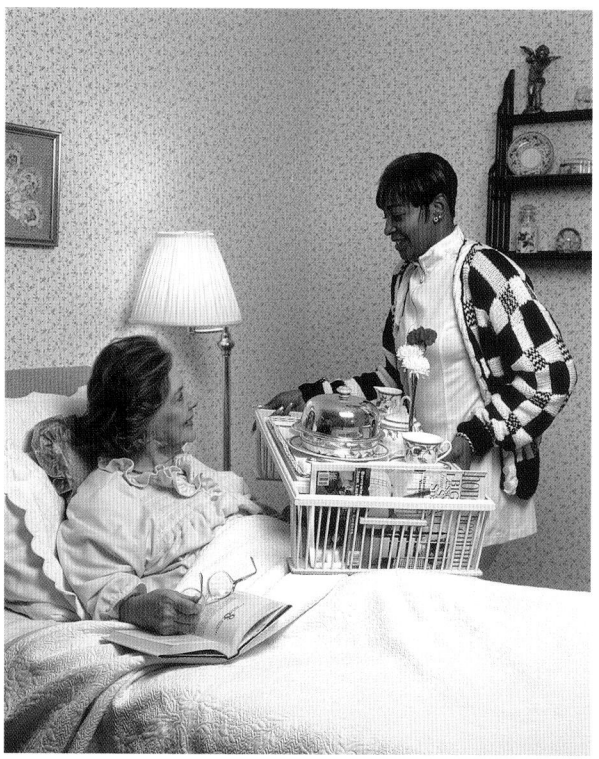

Trained nurses can be hired to take care of the elderly person at home.

FAMILY CONSULTATION

If you plan to care for a parent or grandparent, discuss your plans with members of your extended family, to confirm that you have their support, and which of them will lend a hand when needed. Raise the important subject of finances, how best to cover the costs of home care, and who will contribute to costs as and when necessary.

Consult with the elderly person's doctor and any other medical professionals who have been providing regular care, such as physiotherapists and dieticians. Establish what medical and other routines must be maintained, and whether you can do this yourself, or will need to be supported by regular visits from the relevant community health-workers.

Last, but not least establish, by means of open and frank discussion, whether you have the unqualified support of your spouse and children, particularly if you plan to provide home care to a relative for an extended or indefinite period. The decision will impact on everyone who lives in your home, so ensure that everyone appreciates the adjustments which may be necessary.

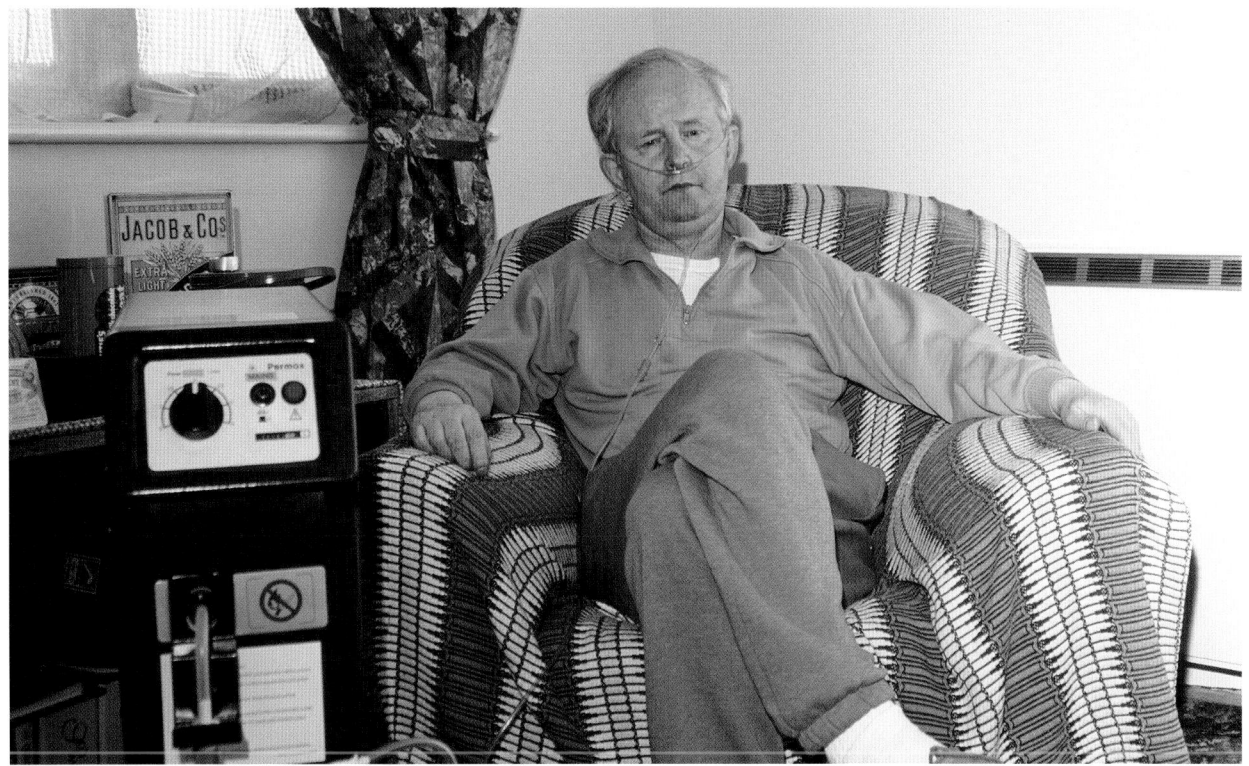

The cost of hiring special equipment must be taken into consideration when you are thinking of inviting an aged family member to come and live with you.

THE PHYSICAL ENVIRONMENT

Some hospitals or frail-care institutions may offer the services of a specially trained community nurse who does home visits and will help you decide how to adapt your home for nursing purposes. If you conduct this exercise on your own, pay attention to:

- **Overall layout**. There should be a bedroom for the sole use of the person being nursed, with easy access to a bathroom and toilet, regardless of whether they are mobile or confined to bed. If the bedroom is in a separate annex, a bell, alarm or intercom should be fitted to allow help to be summoned when necessary.
- **The toilet and bathroom** need to be spacious, so a frail person can manoeuvre themselves easily and safely, particularly if they use walking frames or wheelchairs. Handrails may have to be fitted in the shower or bathtub and alongside the toilet.
- **Staircases**, narrow doorways or poorly lit areas may create obstacles to mobility for physically dis-

abled people or those with poor eyesight. If a wheelchair is used, it is a good idea to borrow one in advance to ensure it can fit through doorways, and that there is room to turn around or manoeuvre in tight spaces.
- **Slippery tiles** and loose mats or rugs can be hazardous to a person unsteady on their feet, and should be avoided.
- **Light switches** should be easily accessible, and there should be a bedside light that can be switched on without getting out of bed.

A home environment which allows the frail person as much free movement as possible will reduce their dependence upon you, and make for a happy arrangement all round.

SPECIAL EQUIPMENT

Medical equipment can be bought or hired, according to the needs of the person you are caring for, and your budget. Items such as beds with side-railings,

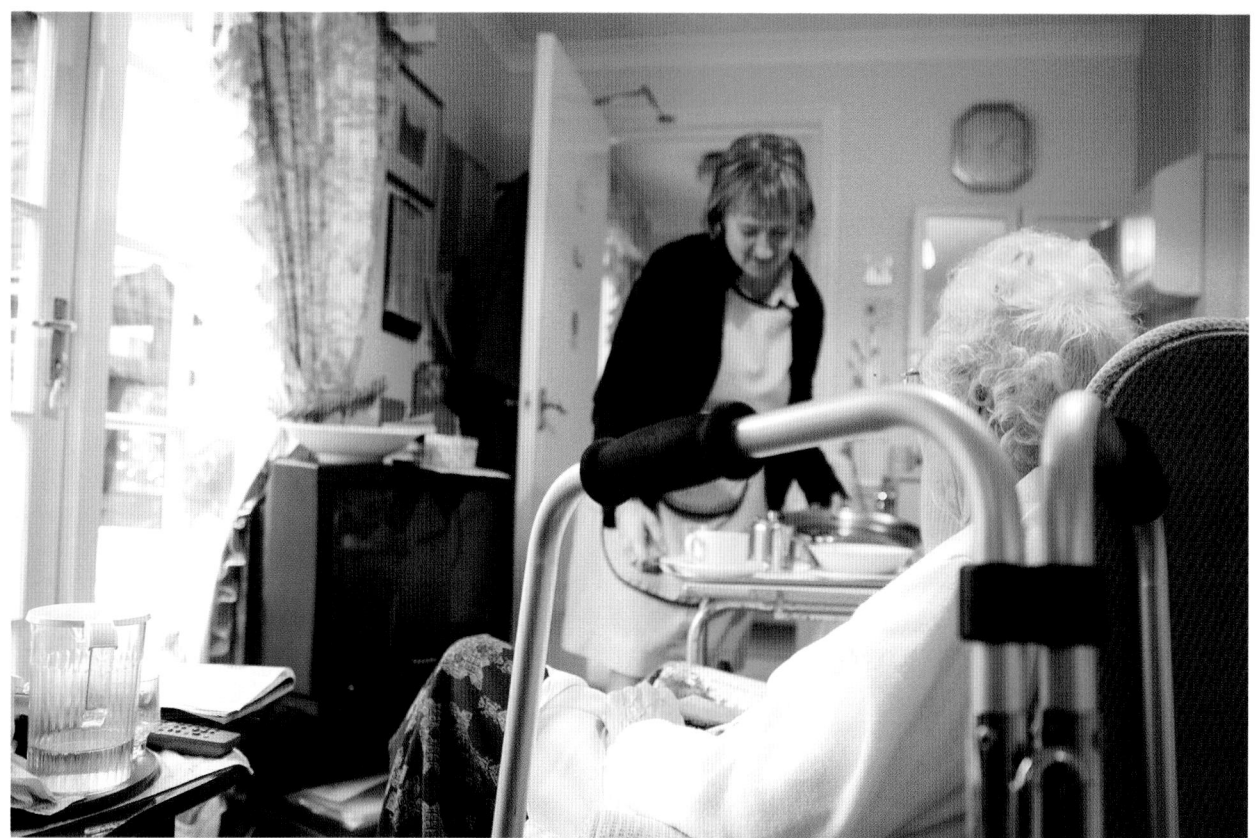

Make sure the patient is kept busy and stimulated not only mentally but also physically. Good nutrition, sunshine, moderate exercise – if possible – and frequent visits will aid their recovery.

walking frames, wheelchairs, commodes and oxygen cylinders are widely available from medical suppliers, while disposable items such as waterproof sheets, urinals and diapers can be obtained from wholesale or retail pharmacies.

Your doctor or community nurse should be able to advise on the type of equipment required for your particular situation.

LIFESTYLE AND ROUTINES

The main advantage of being at home is that it allows the frail, recovering or disabled person to move beyond the role of 'patient', and feel like a normal, dignified member of society despite their medical limitations.

Try to structure your care according to what the disabled or older person essentially needs. Even if it takes Granny two hours to get dressed in the morning, let her do it herself rather than insist on helping. At the same time, be sensitive to the fragile pride of a person who is embarrassed to ask for help. The art is to find a balance between just being available, and knowing when to intervene.

MEDICATION

If the patient is on a strict medication regime, someone must always be available to ensure the correct dosage is taken at the appropriate time. If medication has to be injected, you may require daily visits by a community nurse. Patients who suffer from respiratory illnesses often use a nebulizer throughout the day; they may also need home visits by a physiotherapist who can help relieve chest congestion.

THE BED-BOUND PERSON

A person confined to bed for whatever reason requires special care, in order to prevent the complications of immobility. The areas where you will need to assist are:

- Providing urinals or commodes when necessary, disposing of waste matter and keeping the equipment clean and germ-free.
- Having an adequate supply of fresh bedding, including waterproof undersheets, for a person who is incontinent or partially continent, and having enough hands on deck to change bedding with the person still in the bed.
- Preventing pressure (bed) sores through proper hygiene and skin care, combined with the use of synthetic sheepskins and ensuring regular changes in lying position.
- Providing a varied and interesting diet, which includes a daily portion of fibre to prevent constipation. Inactive people burn up less energy, and therefore require smaller helpings of food. However, unless a special diet is prescribed, there is no reason why they cannot share in the food cooked for the family. Fresh water should always be on hand at the bedside, and fluid intake must be encouraged to prevent the stagnation of urine and the development of bladder infections and kidney stones.
- If meals must be taken in bed, arrange for members of the family to eat with them in the room once or twice a week.

People who are confined to bed, or whose mobility is limited in any way, find that the days become long, tedious, and frustrating. If not adequately occupied during the day, they may simply sleep for long periods, and be restless or sleepless at night, creating a disruption for the whole family. To preserve a normal sleep cycle, provide mental stimulation during the day, with reading matter, radio, television and occasional visitors.

Your family doctor or a community nurse may do house visits for regular checkups.

WILL IT WORK OUT?

The outline of priorities listed in this chapter gives an indication of the substantial investment of your time, energy and money that home care requires. Still, nursing a loved one at home can be a most rewarding experience for all concerned if you have planned carefully and have support from the rest of your family as well as community services.

A person with a chronic illness or a deteriorating mental condition may become more difficult to nurse than originally anticipated, and progressively more demanding on your care. Your own circumstances may not allow you enough time to care for an invalid.

If this happens, do not feel that you are locked into an arrangement, or that you have been defeated. Instead, look carefully at what the invalid requires, discuss the situation with your family doctor, social worker or community nurse and, with their guidance, identify a suitable (and affordable) health provider or institution who can take over. Do not chide yourself for having given up. Award yourself credit for what you have done so far, and don't feel guilty about passing on increasing responsibility when you cannot cope any longer.

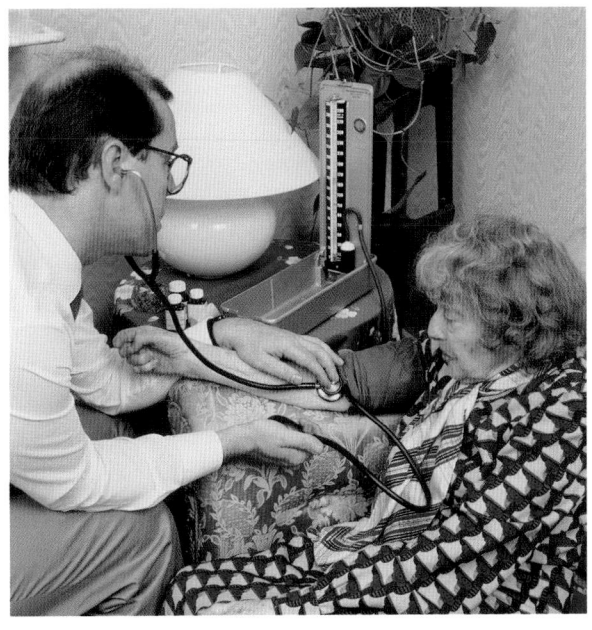

SAFETY AROUND THE HOME

We tend to regard our homes as safe havens, where we are protected from 'danger', but danger comes in many disguises. A home is only as safe as we make it, yet we often take for granted the security afforded by the sense of 'home' and forget to view our living environment in a more rational light.

An important aspect to consider when reviewing the safety of your home is who lives there. A couple with no children or pets may be at ease with open stairwells, a plunge pool and expensive artworks on occasional tables, whereas a family with inquisitive toddlers or active youngsters would be more comfortable in a home that allows the children to explore their surroundings and play freely, yet has sufficient protection to ensure that it is safe for them to do so.

Some home-based emergencies are beyond our ability to prevent, but the vast majority can be prevented. Simple precautions can make the difference between coping with a minor incident or having it turn into a crisis. In these instances, a positive outcome is often determined by your ability to find solutions and then act accordingly. Prevention is not rocket science; the key is common sense. It is also a matter of expecting the unexpected, no matter how improbable it may seem.

IN THIS SECTION

A child-friendly home

Every year thousands of children are treated for injuries sustained in their homes, most of which could have been avoided. We usually run our lives according to what is convenient but, when you have a child in the house, convenience should come after safety, so look at your home through different eyes and put safety first.

There are many things you can do to make your home safer as your child grows from that bundle of fun in the crib to an inquisitive adult in the making. Remember, as your children grow, so will their ability to reach the unreachable, and do what they are not supposed to do. As soon as they can crawl, get down on your hands and knees to see the world from their perspective to decide what he or she might be able to reach. When your child can understand simple instructions, ensure you get across loud and clear the meaning of 'No!' and 'Don't touch!'.

LIVING ROOM AND BEDROOMS

- Make electrical cords and sockets inaccessible and teach children not to touch them.
- Ensure free-standing heaters, electric blankets and hairdryers are in good condition and are used correctly at all times.
- Keep medicines out of your bedside drawer and off low shelves in the cupboard.
- Don't use tablecloths on tables that have lamps, vases or heavy ornaments on them; a child might pull the cloth off, bringing the object down as well.

- Other items that could be pulled over include standing lamps and wobbly bookshelves.
- Install stair guards at the top and bottom of flights of stairs.
- Fit a fire guard in front of an open fireplace.
- Keep children away from heaters (radiators) and circulating fans.
- Buy toys that are suitable for your child's age.
- Ensure young children do not pick up or play with small items like buttons, coins, etc.

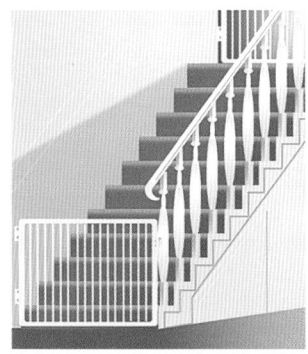
Stair guard

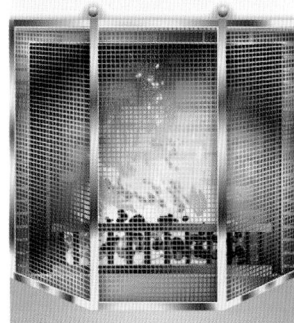
Fire guard

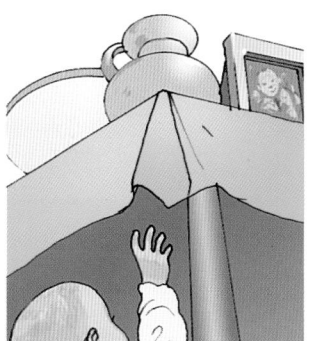
Short tablecloths

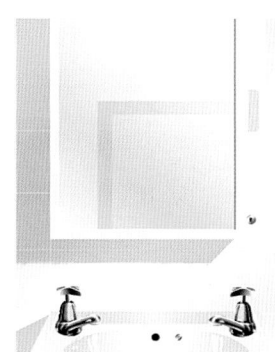
Lock up medicine

THE KITCHEN

The kitchen is not a playground; there is enormous potential for accidents, such as a bad burn or scald, which could scar a child for life.

Wherever possible, use protection devices. Stair guards, for example, not only prevent children going up or down stairs, but can be used to block doorways, to keep them out of the kitchen (a major source of mishaps), or the garage or workshop – an equally rich source of accidents, given the type of tools and chemicals often found there.

When it comes to children's safety, parents need to be consistent. For instance, if your child starts chewing on a length of electrical flex, even though it may be a short off-cut from a connection you have made, stop the child immediately and take the cord away. Why? Because this time it was safe, but next time the child might decide to chew on a wire that is live, with tragic results.

- Keep knives, skewers and other sharp objects out of the way.
- Replace the frayed or damaged electrical cords on appliances.
- Turn pot handles inwards when cooking a meal on top of the stove and ensure that hot dishes are not placed near the edge of the work-surface.
- When you need to use only one or two stove plates or burners, use the rear ones in preference to those at the front.
- If your cupboard doors do not lock, install safety latches, particularly on cupboards or drawers used to store household cleaners and detergents.

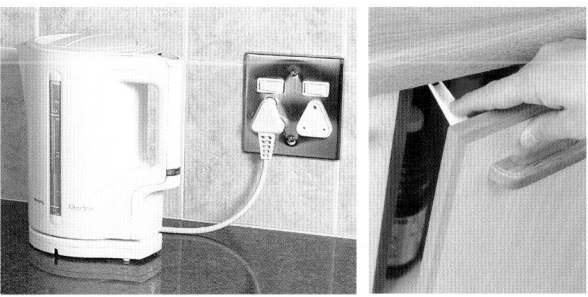

Short electrical cords prevent children from reaching appliances (left). Install child resistant latches in cupboard door (right).

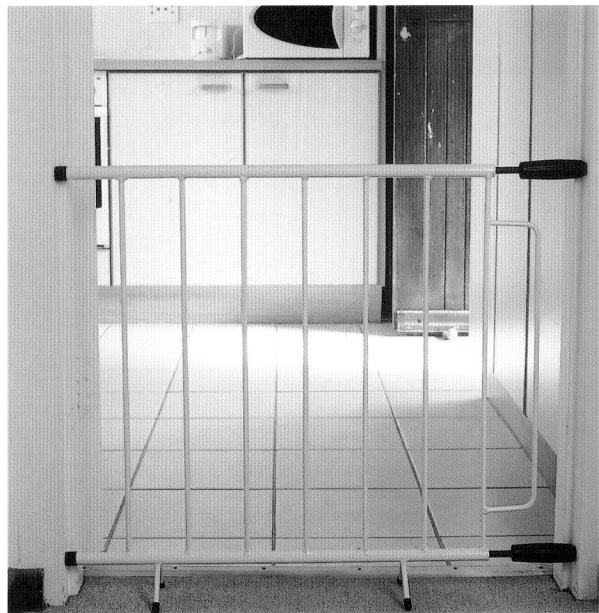

The kitchen is a major source for mishaps. To ensure your toddler's safety store dangerous goods out of reach. When you are not in the kitchen, block access to it with a gate such as the one shown above.

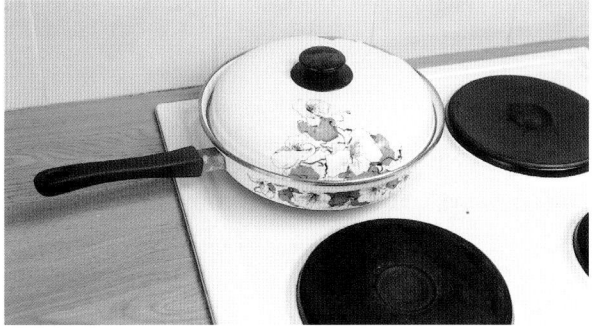

Pot handles must be turned away from the front of the stove where young hands may reach.

- Install thermostatic mixing valves in your bathroom taps to ensure that water is dispensed at a safe temperature. Water with a temperature of 60°C (140°F) can cause severe scalding.
- Always run the cold water into the bath first, and then top up with hot. Test the water temperature with your elbow, or use a thermometer.
- Supervise your toddler's visits to the toilet. A child's weight is biased towards the top half of their body, and if they overbalance head first into the toilet they could drown. For the same reason, use nappy (diaper) buckets with child-resistant lids. Remember, a child can drown in only a couple of centimetres of water.
- Keep medications and toiletries out of their reach, ideally in a lockable cabinet mounted high up against the wall. Try to purchase products stored in child- or tamper-resistant containers designed to resist being opened by small hands.
- Store sharp objects, such as razors, in wall-mounted brackets out of a child's reach.
- All cleaning products should be kept in a locked cupboard. Where possible, buy only containers with tamper-resistant caps.

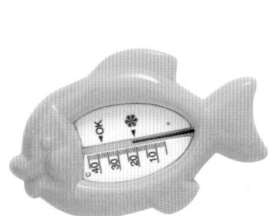
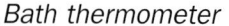

Bath thermometer

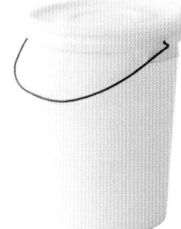

Bucket with tamper-resistant lid.

Child safety

Childproofing should not only concentrate on home and garden, but include car travel and visits to the playground. By taking precautions and adhering to standard safety regulations you can ensure the safety of your child.

SUN GLARE PROTECTION

Other simple, often overlooked, protection devices include hoods or sun visors on carry cots and push chairs, and screens on car windows, all of which help to protect a child's eyes from the sun's glare, and possible damage from UV rays, as well as from windborne dust and other pollutants.

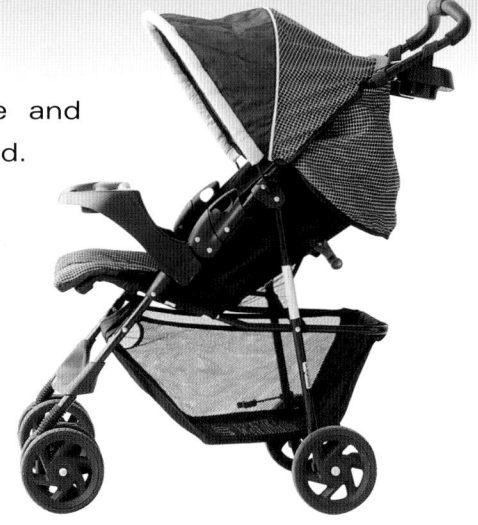

Sun visor and carry net are good ideas. Never hang bags from the handle or the pram could tip.

PLAY AREAS

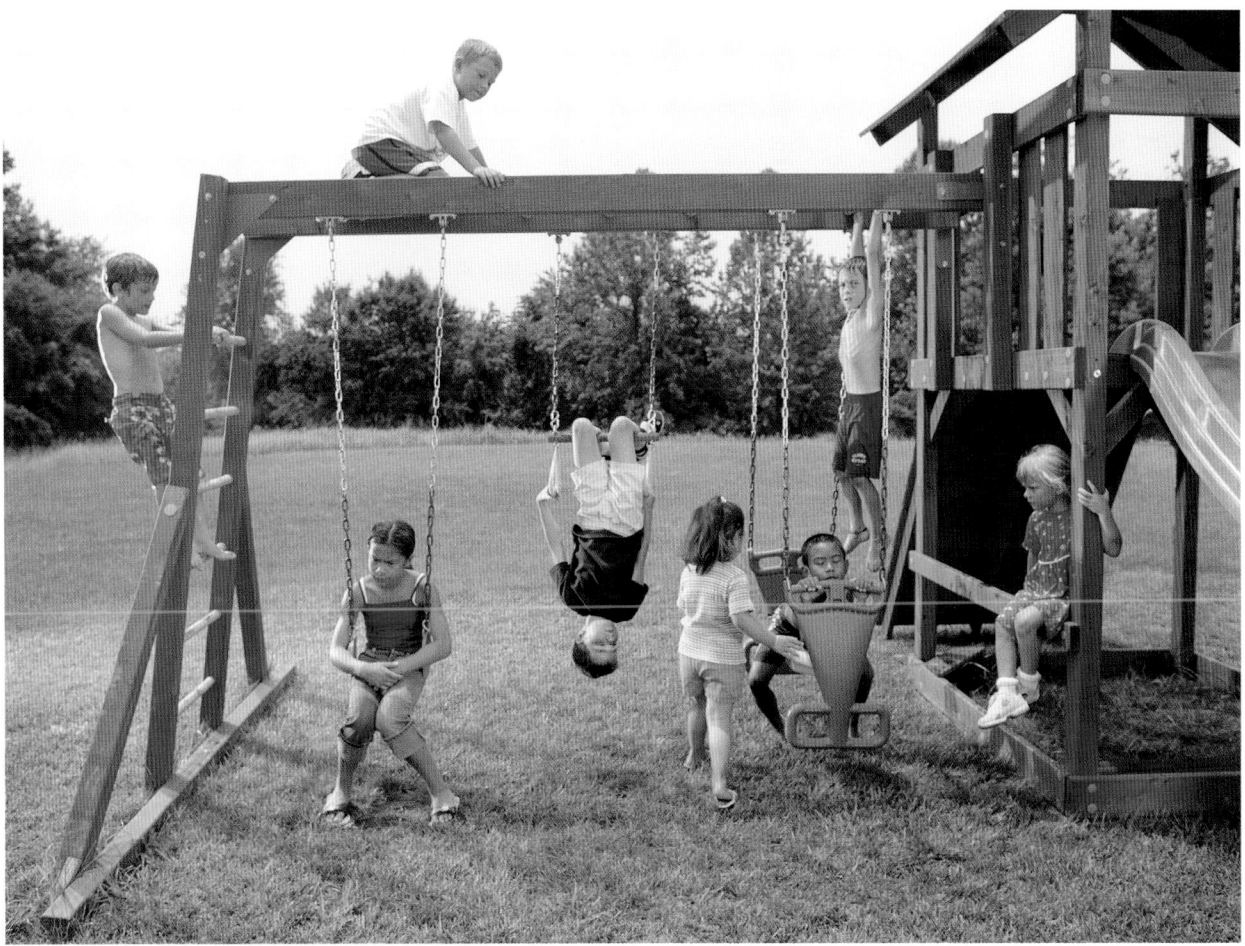

The surface underneath a play structure should be soft to protect against hard falls.

Children learn through play, but they also learn by making mistakes. Parents need to strike a happy balance between protecting their little ones from harm while allowing them enough scope to experiment – even if they end up with a few bumps and bruises, and the odd scratch.

A sturdy wooden climbing frame in the garden is a marvellous idea, not only because children love to clamber over and under things but also because these frames help the child to develop his or her hand-eye co-ordination, strength and imagination.

Do ensure, however, that the ground below the play apparatus is nice and soft – lawn or an area that doubles as a sandpit would be ideal – and that the frame structure is securely fitted into the ground and cannot topple over.

SAFE TRANSPORT

Children are particularly vulnerable in vehicles, no matter whether stationary or not. It is irresponsible and negligent to ignore the safety regulations that dictate that all children up to the approximate age of 11 or 12 should be restrained in specially designed and approved seats. Baby chairs and booster seats provide additional support and a secure safety harness that will ensure minimal injury in the event of an accident and might save your child's life.

In an accident involving a vehicle travelling along at a mere 48kph (30mph), an unrestrained child would be flung around or out of the car with a force up to 50 times greater than its body weight. It makes no difference whether the child is sitting in the back or front seat, or even on the lap of a passenger at the time – it would be crushed instantly or propelled towards the windscreen at a velocity that spells certain disaster.

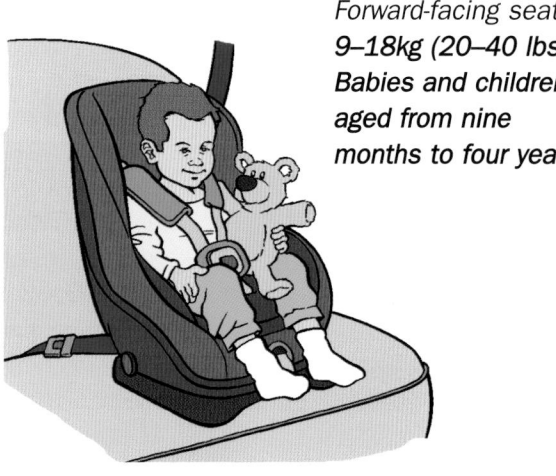

Forward-facing seat: 9–18kg (20–40 lbs). Babies and children aged from nine months to four years.

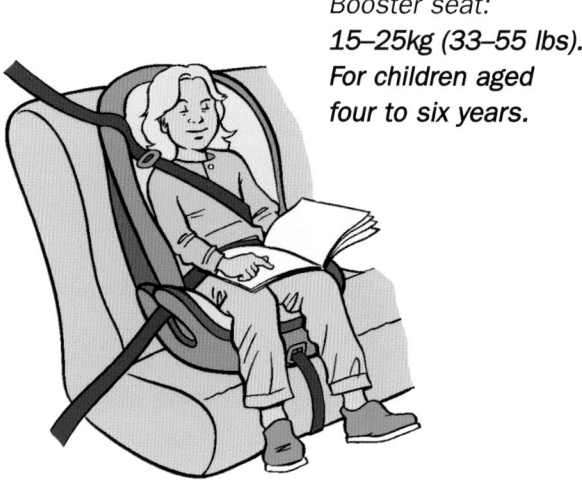

Booster seat: 15–25kg (33–55 lbs). For children aged four to six years.

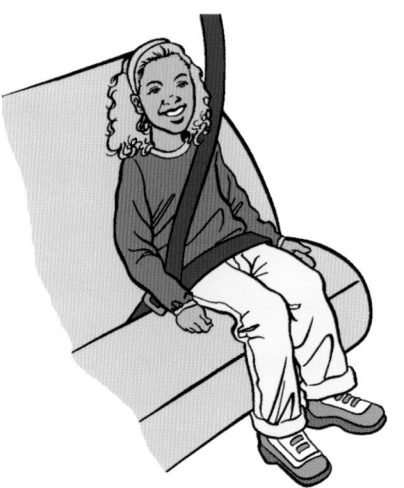

Seat belts are designed to fit around people who are 150cm (5ft) and taller. By the age of 11, your child should be big enough to discard the booster cushion and use the seat belt only.

X DO NOT

- allow a child to stand on a seat or sit on anyone's lap.
- fit a rearward-facing seat on the passenger seat if the car is fitted with front airbags.
- leave a child in the vehicle unattended – not even for a second.
- allow children to play with the vehicle's controls or the ignition key.
- allow children to play with a ball or throw toys about inside the car. The driver could easily be distracted.

Images courtesy of The Royal Society for the Prevention of Accidents (RoSPA)

Assistance for the elderly

The elderly are particularly prone to falls, which frequently result in strains and sprains. The increasing frailty and unsteadiness of old age means that even a minor fall can cause a broken wrist, while a more serious fall could result in a fractured hip.

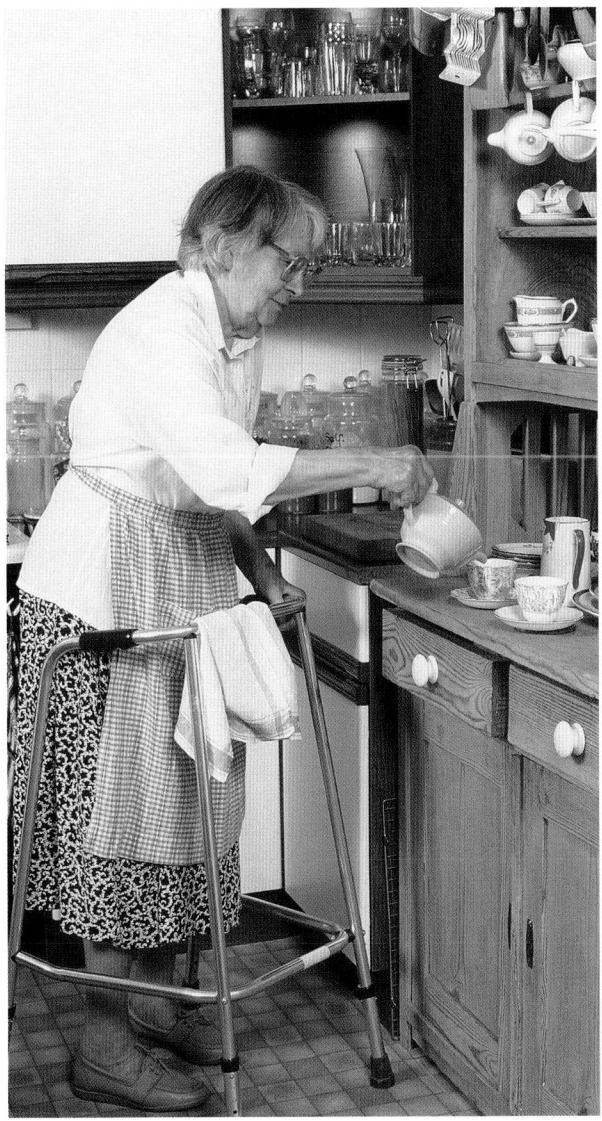

An elderly lady makes use of a zimmer frame to move about in her home.

If you have an elderly person living with you, consider making it easier for them to move around in your home. One simple remedy is to install handrails and non-slip surfaces on stairs and steps, particularly those leading into the garden or outside areas. In cases of extreme frailty, you may also have to consider putting handrails along passageways. Good lighting on stairs is essential, while some form of visual contrast, such as brightly coloured tape or paint to mark the top of each tread, makes it easier to see the edges of steps.

There are many useful aids to assist the elderly (as well as anyone suffering from arthritis or other conditions of limited mobility): scissor-grabs help to pick up anything they have dropped; a hook enables them to open and close windows; tap extensions make it easier to open and close a tap (faucet); and special chairs enable them to get in and out of the bath or shower.

If a wheelchair is going to become a necessity, you will probably have to make a number of adjustments, such as constructing a wheelchair ramp for access to and from the house, and moving furniture around to allow enough space for manoeuvring.

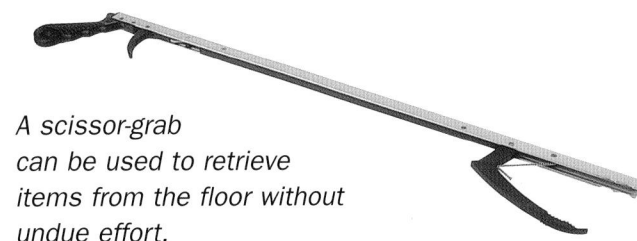

A scissor-grab can be used to retrieve items from the floor without undue effort.

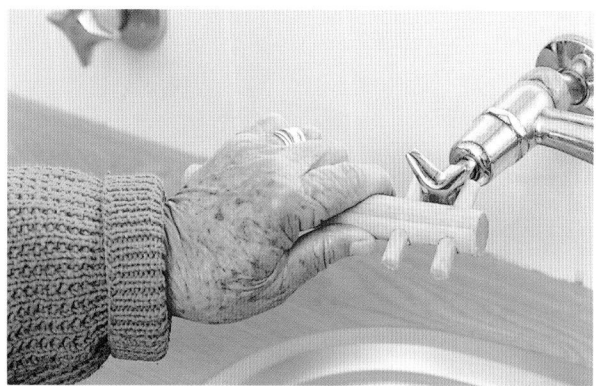

A simple tool like this makes it easier for old hands to open and close taps.

HANDY HINTS

- Position kettles, microwaves and hotplates so that the aged can reach them more easily.
- Overfull kettles are harder to lift, and may be dropped, so use just enough water.
- Remove loose mats and rugs, as it is easy to slip, or catch a foot and fall.
- Install good lighting in passageways, shaded exterior areas and stairwells. Ensure lights leading to the bathroom are accessible.
- Move obstacles such as occasional tables, large plant pots and small items of furniture, allowing a clear route to and from doorways.

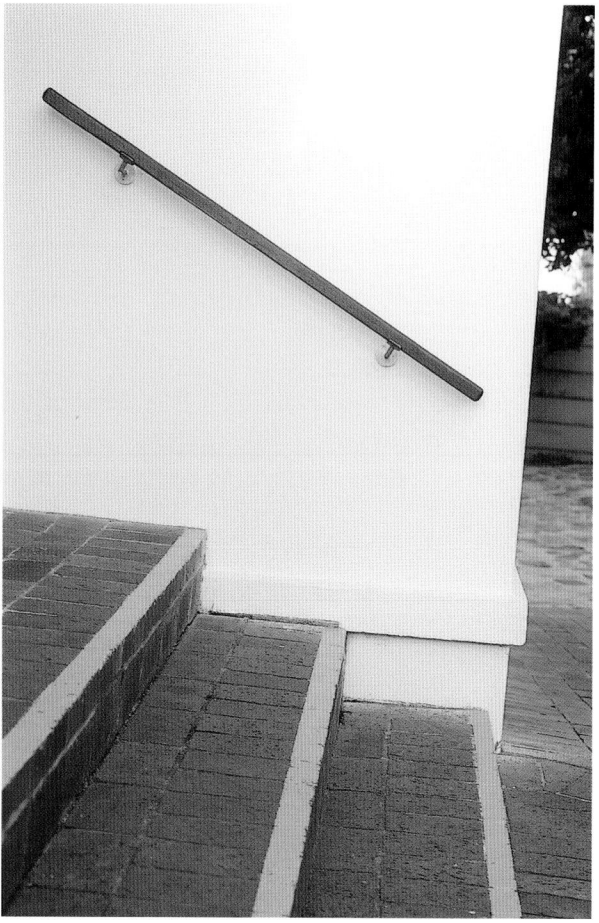

Handrails and brightly painted edges make it easier to see and negotiate a flight of steps.

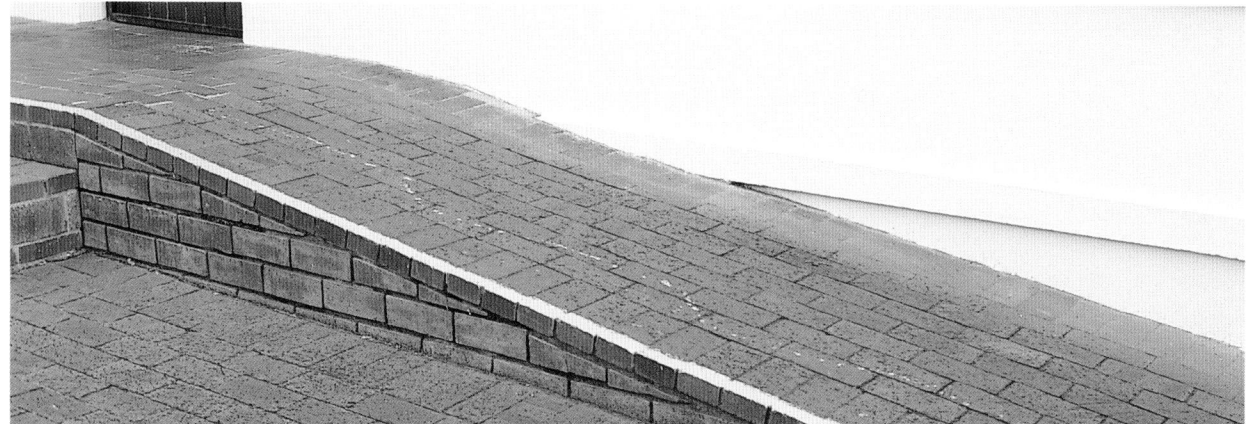

Painting a prominent yellow strip on the edge of a wheelchair ramp makes it more visible, particularly at night or in poor light. Any ramp for wheelchairs needs to have a gentle gradient (slope).

Fire precautions

Of all the disasters that can strike a home and family, fire ranks as one of the most traumatic, not only because of its danger to life and risk of injury, but also because it destroys so comprehensively. However, there are some preventative steps you can take:

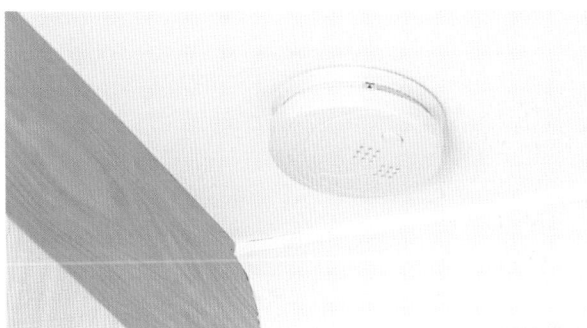

- Install smoke detectors as suggested by the manufacturers. Test the alarms, and check and replace the batteries regularly.
- Buy fire extinguishers and mount them near the doorways of areas most at risk.
  - Keep a container of bicarbonate of soda close to the stove. Sprinkled on flames it will extinguish a small flare-up quickly and effectively.
  - Ensure all electrical fittings, wiring and appliances are in good order and replace as they become worn or frayed.
  - Never run electric cords under carpets or rugs. In time, foot traffic can damage their insulation, resulting in a short circuit which could cause a fire.
- Select non-flammable materials when choosing carpets, drapes (curtains) and furniture.
- Keep clothing and other flammable items well away from incandescent bar heaters (electric fires or radiators) and open flame gas heaters.
- Use a fire guard in front of an open fire.
- Use dry coal or anthracite. If coal or anthracite is wet when you add it to the fire, the moisture in it turns to steam, builds up pressure and fragments

are blown off. While these can mark your carpet, they might also cause a fire, or an injury if a piece lands in someone's eye.

Smoke detectors are essential. Mount them outside the kitchen in the hall, on the landing, as well as in the garage and workshop.

TAKE NOTE

It is essential that you learn to use your fire extinguisher correctly and that you have it checked regularly to ensure that it won't let you down in an emergency.

CAUTION

- Never fight a fire unless it is small and you are confident that you can get it under control safely and quickly.
- This is not the time to take risks. If the fire is too big then: **get out, stay out and call the fire brigade**.
- Never use water on a fire caused by an electrical fault. If the power is still on, you run the risk of electrocution.
- Never use water on a fire caused by liquid fuel. Most flammable liquids float on water, you will simply spread the problem.

FIGHTING FIRES

The most important point to consider is that a fire extinguisher is only as good as the person who is using it. **Let everyone in your house learn how to use the extinguisher and have it checked regularly so that it won't let you down in an emergency**.

When it comes to choosing a fire extinguisher, it is important to consider where it might be used. Dry powder (chemical) extinguishers are best as they can be used on fires fuelled by wood, paper, textiles or flammable liquids, as well as those caused by an electrical short circuit.

- Buy two small, portable extinguishers instead of a single large one that might be unwieldy. Position the extinguishers strategically in different areas of the home, such as at the entrance to the garage and near the kitchen.
- A fire blanket, which is simply dropped on to the fire to smother the flames, can be useful.

FIRE DRILL

- Turn off the power, gas line or whatever else might be fuelling the fire.
- Close all windows or doors leading to the area where the fire is, in order to avoid fanning the flames and to deprive the fire of oxygen.
- Try to smother the fire with a non-flammable material, such as a fire blanket.
- Aim a dry powder extinguisher at the base of the fire, not at the flames.
- If a frying pan ignites, cover it with a large lid or wooden board to smother the flame. Do not throw water over the fire – fat floats on water and you risk spreading the flames and causing more damage. Do not lift the lid to see whether the fire is out. Switch off the stove and leave the pan or pot in place for at least 30 minutes.

If a pot catches fire, simply smother the flames by placing a lid over the pot.

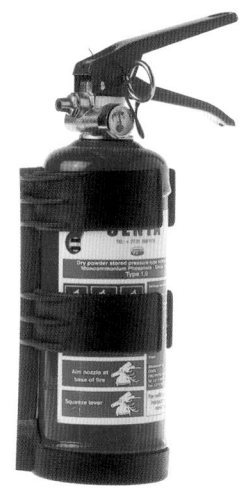
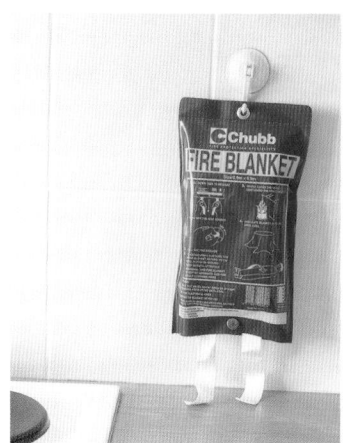

Dry powder fire extinguishers must be checked regularly.

A fire blanket is best kept near the stove area and is thrown over a fire to smother the flames.

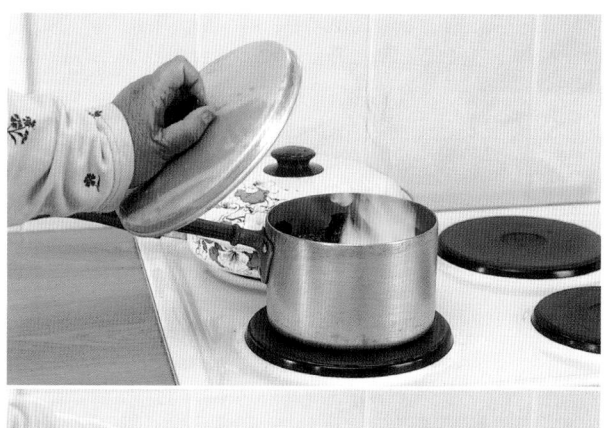
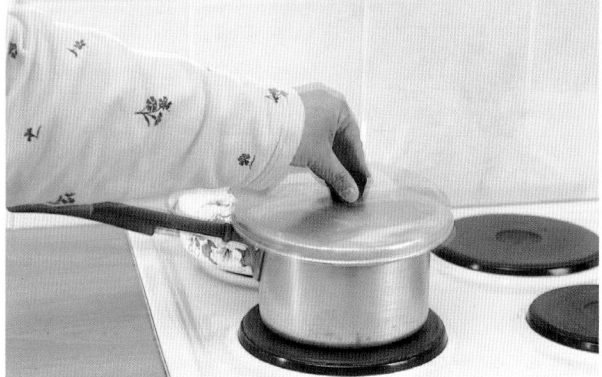

Don't be electrocuted

Electric power is a wonderful thing – right up to the second where you become the conduit between the source and the ground. Many tragic home accidents are due to accidental electrocution and there is a general call to revise the legislation governing DIY electrical work so that it must in future be inspected and passed by a qualified controller. If you are not familiar with how electricity works, get a professional to do all your installations or repairs. Assuming you are capable of carrying out simple electrical tasks, however, here are some basic rules:

HANDY HINTS

- Switch off an electrical appliance at the wall socket and unplug it before dismantling it or probing it with anything.
- As you dismantle the unit, make a careful note of what connection goes where; getting it wrong on re-assembly could turn the unit into a killer.
- Before doing any work on your home's fixed wiring (a socket for instance), let everyone in the home know what you are doing and then:

- Turn off the main power supply at the distribution board and place a large 'Do not touch' notice over the main board.
- Leave a light switched on, connected to an extension cord if necessary, and place it next to you so that, if anyone ignores your instructions, the light will come on and perhaps give you the split second warning that could save your life. An alternative is to leave a radio or TV on and turned up to full volume. You might deafen your neighbours for a minute or two, but it will be worth it.

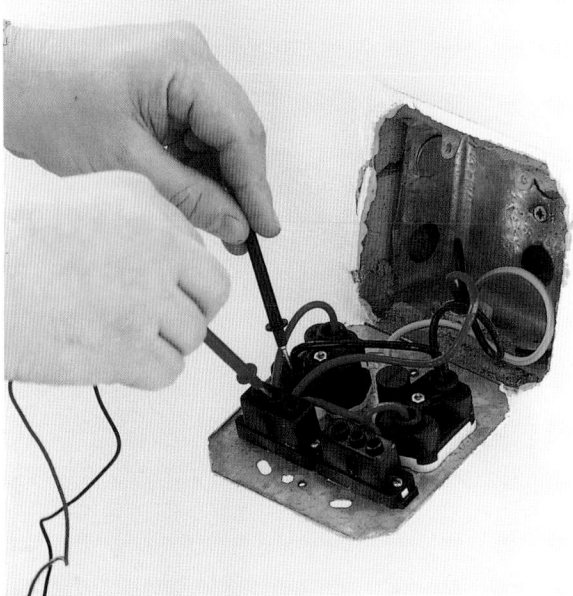

Test an electrical socket before working on it; taking two precautions too many is better than taking one too few.

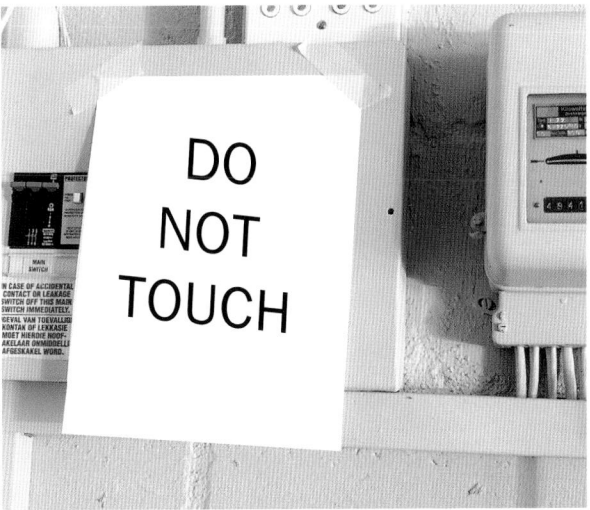

Use a large, clear sign on the distribution board to alert your family while you work on your home's electrical system, and make sure that everyone knows why the power is disconnected.

SAFETY OUTDOORS

Homes begin and end at the front gate, not at the front door, so it is important that when we focus on safety in the home, we give consideration to the exterior environment as well. Whether your backyard is only a few metres across or large and spacious, it often fulfils a variety of functions. Driveways and garages, sheds and workshops, play areas and patios all present their own set of potential dangers. Then, of course, there is the garden, which offers up a whole range of things to watch out for, from poisonous plants to the safe storage and use of insecticides and pesticides.

Home maintenance can also come under the general theme of exterior safety, as neglecting to repair or renovate in time can lead to deterioration. In the case of a rotten roof, this could necessitate costly repairs, but if a fence is left to fall apart, a child could easily slip through and wander onto a busy road. By thinking ahead and taking simple preventative steps, we can minimize the risk and ensure that our entire home environment, inside and out, is safe at all times.

IN THIS SECTION

Nonslip paved surfaces

Paved surfaces, such as paths and patios, are hard-wearing and virtually maintenance-free. There are many different surfacing materials, from rustic brick through stone chips to polished marble or travertine, all of which vary in their natural degree of unevenness and slipperyness when wet. Covered porches, patios or verandas are often given a surface treatment that blends with the internal décor, only to discover that their highly polished floor becomes treacherous when it gets wet. It can be an expensive exercise to relay a surface so, if you are installing a new path or patio, think carefully about what it will be used for. Outdoor living areas and paths leading to and from the house should be even, with a nonslip finish, whereas driveway surfaces might need to offer some traction, particularly if your area is prone to heavy rain or snowfalls.

POOL SURROUNDS

Swimming pool environments are designed for fun and play, but wet surfaces can be slippery. Apart from the bruises, sprains and other injuries that can result from falls, a major concern is someone falling into the water. The best solution is to forbid your children to run around the pool and to ensure that no one ever uses the pool alone or unsupervised.

· Ban everyone from diving or jumping into the shallow end of a swimming pool.
· When building a new pool, ensure that the coping (edge) provides an easy-to-grip handhold for even the smallest hands.
· Select a good quality, long-lasting nonslip surface for the surrounds – a pebble-dashed type of surface is worth considering. Take time to make your choice, as the right one could save you a great deal of heartache.

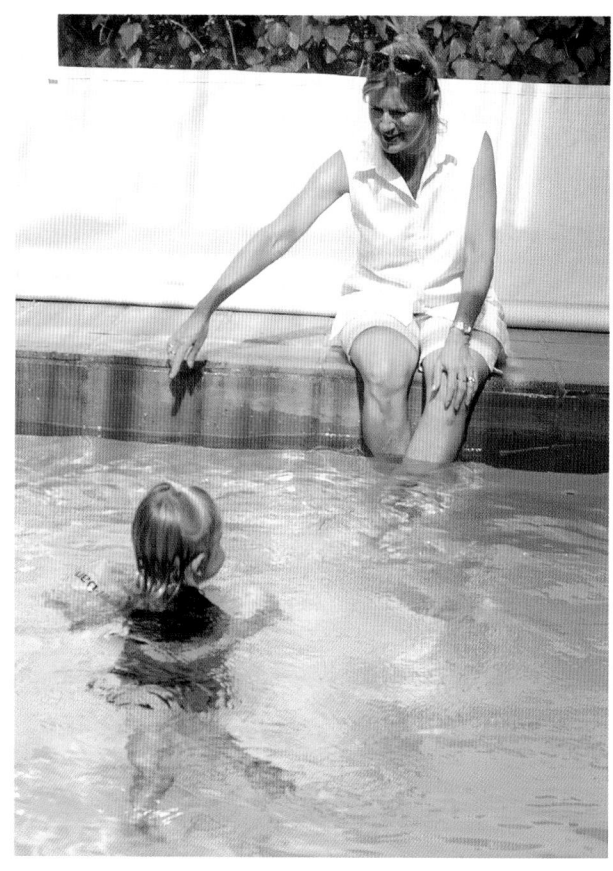

Pool paving should be made of nonslip material and have coping that is easy to grasp .

PATHS AND PAVING

REMOVING MILDEW AND MOSS FROM PAVING SURFACES

Mildew is a plant disease and moss a plant species, but both can cause some paving surfaces to become very slippery, particularly in wet weather or when there is dew. There are purpose-made products designed to eradicate mildew but these can take some time to work. For quick results, hire or buy a high-pressure water cleaner and blast the deposits away. Spreading coarse gravel over the worst areas will provide a temporary nonslip surface.

While velvety moss can look attractive between paving stones, for safety's sake, it is best to limit its spread to the edges of paths, or less-used parts of the garden. Gardeners tend to wear wellingtons or sturdy footwear that will not slip easily, but give mossy paths a miss when you are wearing 'everyday shoes'.

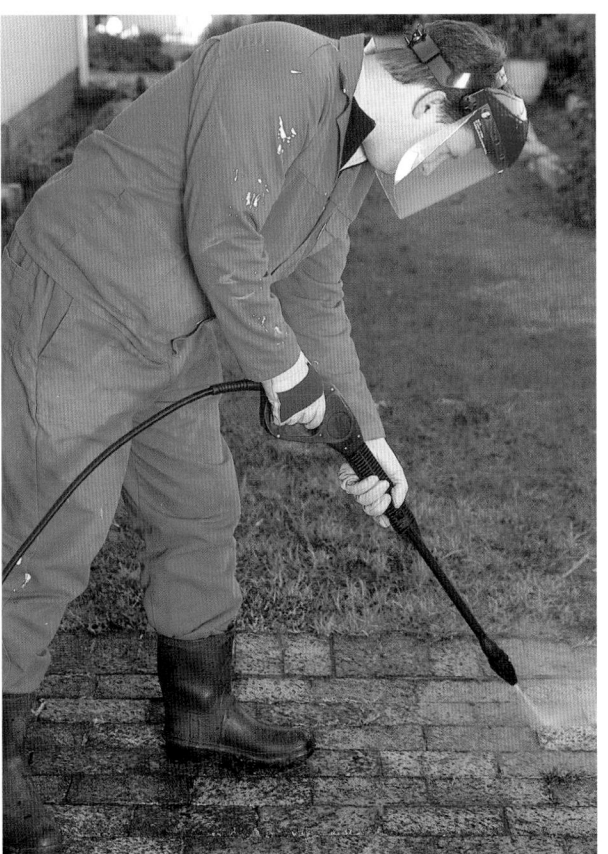

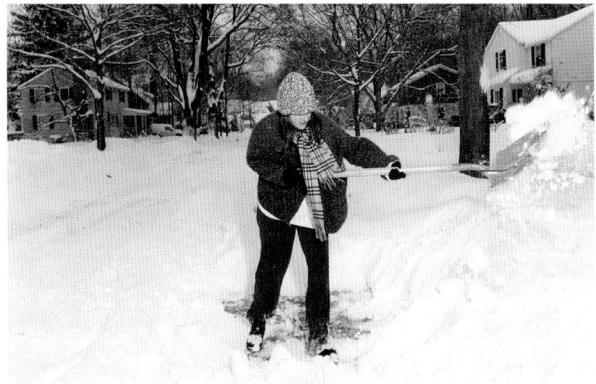

Removing snow from a pathway.

CLEARING SNOW-BOUND PATHS

The onset of winter often means having to deal with snow. If your home has a driveway or a path leading to the street, you'll have to invest in equipment to keep the path cleared and safe to walk on. A good-quality shovel is useful for clearing heavy falls of snow, and a broom will handle a light dusting. Motorized 'snowblowers' are a more costly option, but get the job done quickly.

Fresh powder snow is light and easy to clear; wet snow is always heavier. If you let snow lie in the hope that the sun will melt it, you may find that a thick layer of ice has formed underneath. The difference between day and night temperatures can lead to the formation of a thin layer of ice ('black ice'), which can lead to falls, especially if it is covered by fresh snow. Sand or fine grit scattered over your cleared path or driveway will prevent accidents and give tyres a better grip.

Salt can also be used to thaw ice and snow, but the use of salt can have negative consequences, such as salt build-up in your garden. Be sure to find out if municipal regulations in your area permit the use of salt.

A high-pressure hose is an effective way to blast moss and mildew from paved surfaces.

Safety on the roof

The greater a roof's slope (pitch), the more dangerous it is. When in doubt, get the professionals in, and do not attempt to work on a high (double-storey) or steeply pitched roof yourself. If your roof is low, flat or has a gentle pitch, you can undertake simple repairs or maintence, providing you observe basic precautions and have a stable ladder. For more intricate work or repairs that cannot be done relatively quickly, it is safer to hire a tower scaffold so that you can stand on it and work from a fixed platform.

Tie yourself up there so that, if you do slip, the worst injury you can sustain is a graze and some wounded pride. To do this, throw a length of stout rope over the roof, more or less where you will be working, and secure it on the opposite side to a sturdy, stationary anchor, such as a large tree or patio column. Once you are on the roof, wrap the free end of the rope around your waist and secure it with a good knot. If you have a safety harness, tie it to that. Adjust the length of the rope as you work, but be careful not to trip over it or become entangled in it.

HANDY HINTS

- Begin by sweeping the work area before starting the repair job – even dry debris can be deadly and cause you to slip and fall.
- Wear nonslip footwear that fastens securely; slip-on sandals are a no-no.
- Warn others to stay away from the eaves – a dropped tool can cause a serious injury.
- When on the roof, put your tools on a nonslip mat so that they are secure.
- Use a rope to pull heavy tools up (when on a ladder, use both hands for this).
- Stay clear of overhead power or phone lines.
- If roofing material cannot take your full weight, step along the line of the roofing timbers or place boards across them to spread your weight.
- Do not go onto the roof while the surface is wet from dew or rain, or if there is any chance of rain or a storm with lightning.
- Do not work on roofs with a slope (pitch) greater than 30°.

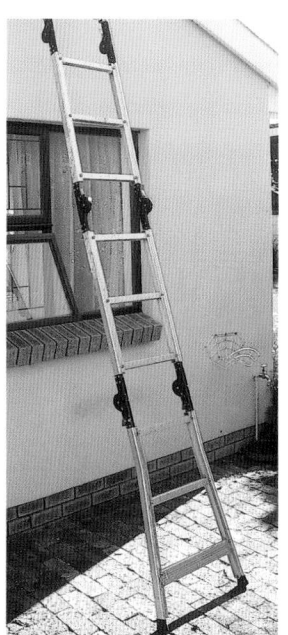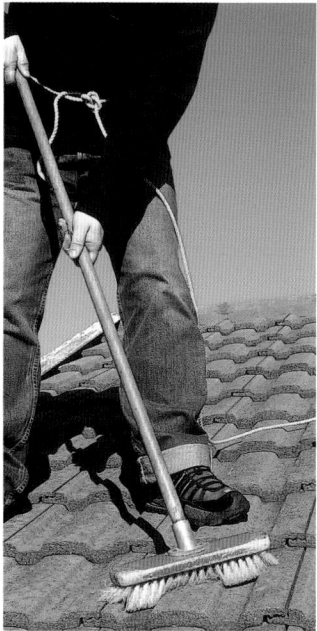

Make sure your ladder is at a safe angle (left). Sweep away any debris that may be slippery (right).

LADDER KNOW-HOW

Many gardening and DIY jobs require the use of a stepladder which should be steady, secure and in good condition. If you intend working on the roof, or have a double-storey house, there will be times when an extension ladder is required. Careless use of ladders can result in falls, with sometimes serious consequences, but taking a few simple steps before you ascend can minimize the chance of an accident.

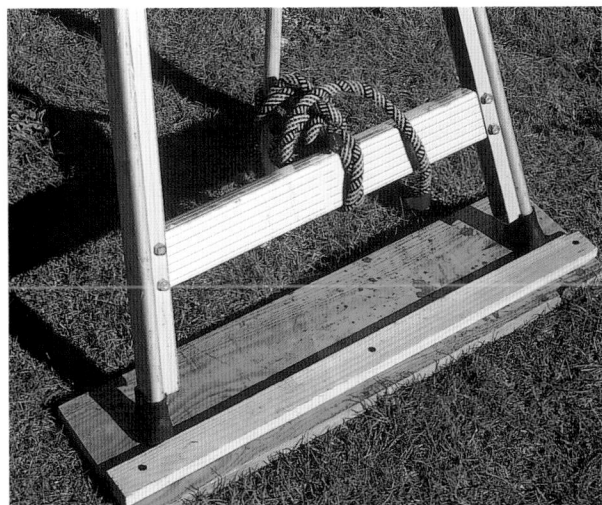

A secure base will prevent the ladder's feet from slipping away.

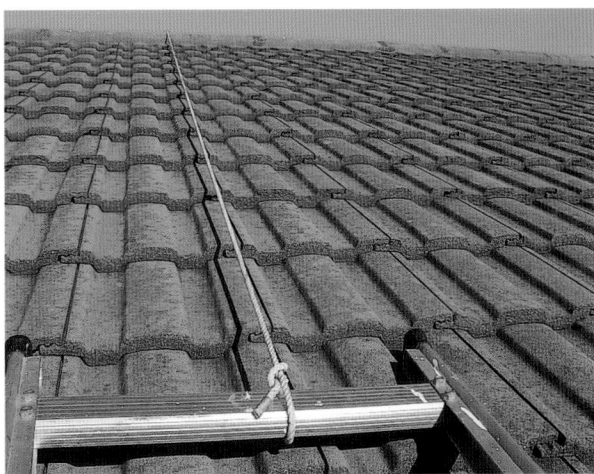

Secure the top rung of the ladder over the roof.

- When using an extension ladder, keep the angle between it and the wall at about 75°.
- To stop the ladder slipping, drive a stake into the ground between the wall and the ladder's feet and tie the bottom rung to the stake. If the ground is soft, rest the ladder on a plank to provide extra support (*see* left).
- Climb the ladder a couple of rungs. If you are satisfied it will not slip backwards, continue. At the top, tie the top rungs to a secure stay, such as a roof truss. You can now climb up the ladder without the fear that it might slide away from under you, or fall away from the wall.
- Wear closed shoes, not loose or slip-on footwear when mounting a ladder.
- Don't mount a ladder if the soles of your shoes are wet due to rain or heavy dew.

MAKING NONSLIP LADDER TREADS

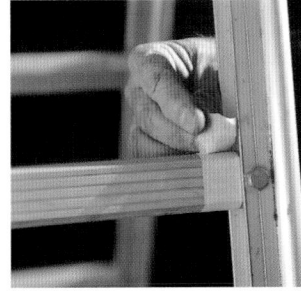

1. *Mask off areas that do not need paint.*

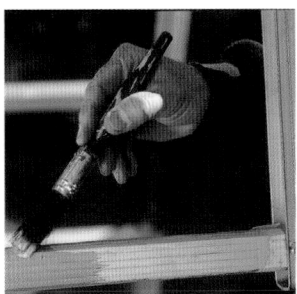

2. *Use bright paint for visibility.*

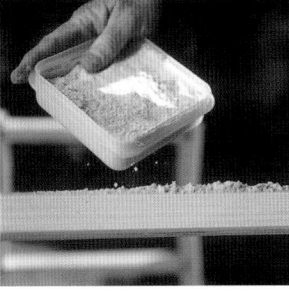

3. *Add coarse sand to wet paint.*

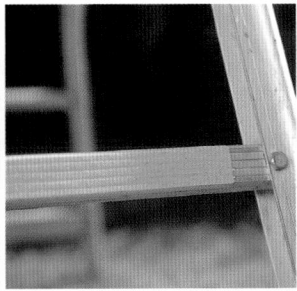

4. *Finish with a final coat of paint.*

Safety in the garage or workshop

The garage, shed or workshop is a place just begging for accidents to happen, filled as it is with sharp and potentially dangerous tools and materials. While regular DIYers tend to be careful and safety conscious, there are many potential hazards which can harm the uninitiated, so keep the garage or workshop securely locked when you are not using it.

HANDY HINTS

- Always wear protective gear when using cutting tools. Safety glasses or goggles are a must, and heavy-duty gloves are preferable. Depending on what you are doing, you may also require some form of ear protection.
- Use a Residual Current Device (RCD). It will cut the electricity if there is a fault or if a cable is accidentally cut.
- Wear clothing that covers most of your body and limbs (overalls). Do not wear loose-fitting garments with tassles or tie-fastenings that could catch in machinery.
- Make sure the lighting is adequate. A single, low-wattage overhead bulb can cast awkward shadows, particularly at night. If necessary, use a portable light on an extension cable to illuminate the item you are working on. If you spend a lot of time in the workshop, consider installing a decent lighting system.
- If you have long hair, tie it back. Clip back a long fringe so it can't flop in your eyes. Before you start, move into your working position to check whether your hair could get in the way.
- Keep children, pets and other distractions out of the workplace when you are busy.
- Never operate tools, power or otherwise, if you have consumed alcohol or are on a course of medication that makes you drowsy.
- Never operate power tools if you are angry or stressed as you will not be thinking straight.

- Ensure all electrical connections are sound and never overload fuses, circuits, motors or outlets. Never replace a blown fuse with one of a higher rating.
- Before using any tools or appliances, check all wiring for frayed ends or worn insulation.
- Never smoke near flammable materials or while using aerosol paints or sprays.
- If doing anything involving heat – welding for instance, do it away from where your flammable materials are stored.

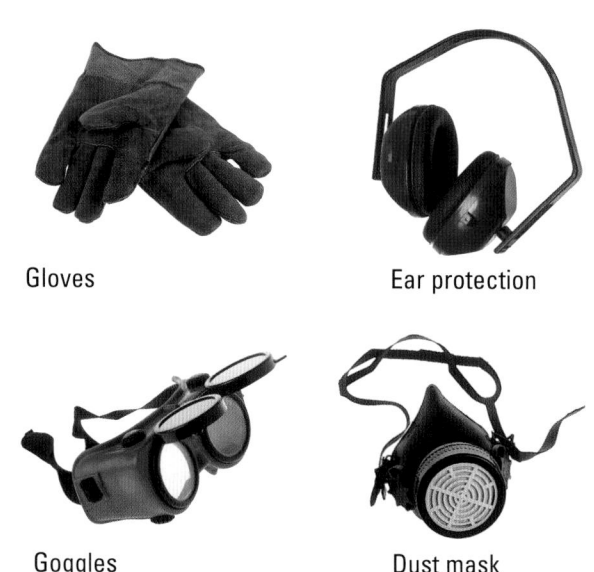

Gloves

Ear protection

Goggles

Dust mask

It is essential that you wear protective gear while working with cutting tools.

- Store flammable materials (such as paints, solvents and gas cylinders) so that you can get them out in a hurry. A handy solution is to mount a shelf, rack or storage bin on casters (an old bookshelf works well); in an emergency you can push the whole lot out of danger in one fell swoop.
- Keep your workshop tidy and clear of debris such as wood shavings, oily rags and used solvents in open containers. Contact your local authority about the proper disposal of chemicals or contaminated items, particularly those that may be harmful to the environment.
- If working with materials that produce fumes, work outside, or at least in the doorway. Using a fan to blow fumes away is an additional precaution.
- Ensure your work-piece is securely clamped into place before picking up any tool, particularly a power tool.

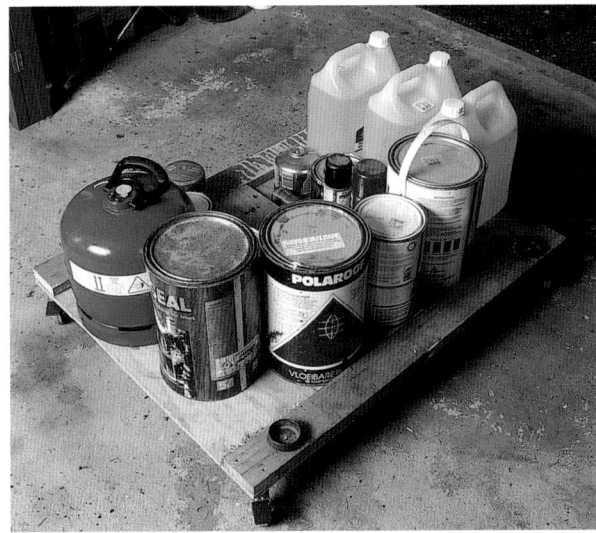

Store containers with flammable materials on an easily moveable trolley.

POWER TOOLS

Power tools such as drills, angle grinders and band saws are great labour-savers, but they can be deadly if misused. As they are designed to facilitate many DIY tasks, they make short work of any material to which they are applied, be it wood, metal, etc. The trouble is that most construction materials are much harder and more resilient than flesh and bone, which means that power tools can cut flesh like a hot knife through butter, and a great deal more painfully.

- Use power tools as intended by the manufacturers and for the purpose for which they were designed.
- Learn to use each tool before getting down to working with it.
- One basic rule is to hold a power tool properly and adopt the right stance before beginning to work – problems can arise if you stumble or trip.
- Before you begin to work,

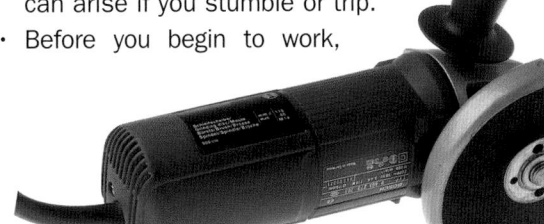

An angle grinder

clear the work area of anything that could distract you. If you get distracted, stop, and switch off the power tool. Do not work while carrying on a conversation, reprimanding the kids, or helping to decide what's for dinner.
- Don't mess about with the safety features. If a guard is provided, leave it in place; do not adapt it to keep it clear of the work piece.
- Ensure the cable is behind the machine. Work away from, never towards, the cable.
- High-quality power tools are well insulated, but don't use them outdoors in the rain, or while standing in a puddle on the floor.
- If you overload the tool and get that 'electric smell', run the machine under no load for a few seconds to allow the fan to cool down the mechanism.
- Never change an accessory, such as a blade or drill bit, without turning off and unplugging the machine.
- Secure the work-piece before you start work.
- Wear suitable protective gear for eyes, ears and face – the fine debris some tools throw out can cause health problems later in life.
- Tie-up long hair, and remove chains, bracelets or rings that could catch on parts of the power tool.
- Unplug power tools when you finish, clean and check them before putting them away.

Garden tools and equipment

In our attempts to create the perfect garden, we use a variety of pesticides, insecticides and weedkillers to combat pests or plant diseases. Many garden chemicals are poisonous and must be stored safely, out of reach of children and pets. Where possible, seek environmentally friendly alternatives and plant in such a way that natural organic defences, such as ladybirds (ladybugs), other insects and birds, reduce the need for artificial intervention.

HANDY HINTS

STORING GARDEN CHEMICALS

- Keep substances in their original containers, but check every so often to ensure that the packaging is in good condition and properly sealed. If a carton tears or breaks, transfer the contents to a new container and label it clearly. Dispose of the old one as laid down in your local ordinances.
- Some products are packed in cardboard boxes, which can deteriorate over time. Keep the contents, in the original packaging, in a larger container that seals (such as a plastic box or big zip-lock bag). Then, if the cardboard does disintegrate, there won't be any spillage.
- Treat garden chemicals as you would medicines, and discard any that have reached their expiry date, as they are likely to become less effective, and may even become unsafe.
- Store corrosive garden chemicals on lower shelves secured behind child resistant locks, rather than higher up. If one of them develops a leak, the contents will not flow over the other stored items. At best, boxes and labels might be damaged; at worst, the chemicals could combine and create a greater hazard.

Store poisons in a locked container.

USING GARDEN CHEMICALS

- When spraying plants, wear protective gear to cover your nose and mouth, and keep children and pets away from the area.
- Don't spray when there is a breeze, even a light one; as the spray will disperse and fine droplets could be carried far enough away to land in a person's or pet's eyes or food, or in a swimming pool or water feature.
- Check your garden on a regular basis and act as soon as you notice a problem with pests. Ignoring insects or pests could lead to your garden being overrun, instigating the trouble and expense of large-scale spraying.

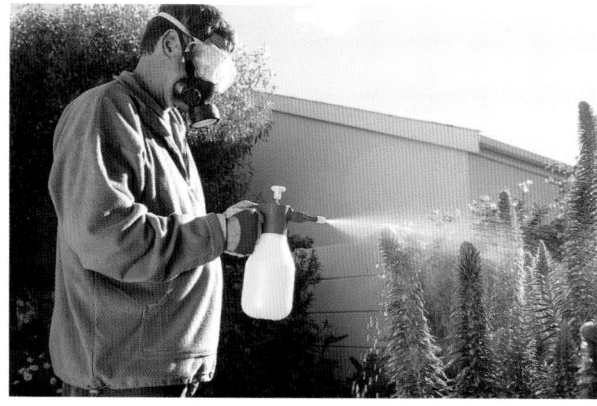

Wear protective goggles and a mask when spraying chemicals, and choose a windstill day.

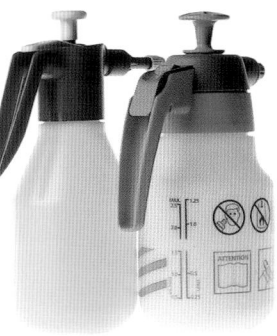

- Use the right spray. If it is not formulated for the pest in question, you'll be wasting time and money. Ensure you fully understand the instructions and keep any instruction leaflet that accompanies the product – the label on the container might not carry all the information you require.
- Always mix the formulation exactly as recommended in the instructions. Stronger is unlikely to be better and you can create more problems than you are solving.
- Mix sufficient spray solution for just a single application, as old mixtures are ineffective and could be dangerous. You might also forget what you have used, and could end up making a mistake the next time.
- Keep two clearly marked spray bottles – one for weedkillers and the other for insecticides. Clean each spray bottle thoroughly after use, as even a small chemical residue could contaminate a new solution.
- Never use empty garden sprayers for any other purpose. To discard a glass container, wrap it in a layers of newspaper and dispose of it safely. Puncture plastic containers and dispose of them safely as well.

USING GARDEN TOOLS SAFELY

Always use a Residual Current Device (RCD) when you operate power tools. Also bear in mind that the cutting parts of edge trimmers and electric or petrol-driven lawn mowers can do a lot of damage if they come loose. Spades and forks can do a fair share of damage and even small items, such as hand-shears or secateurs, can inflict a nasty wound if they are used carelessly, or dropped on a bare foot.

Never leave garden tools lying around when you have finished working with them. Take a few extra minutes to clean or oil them and put them away securely. In that way they'll be ready for the next time and you will also reduce the risk of injury in an unnecessary accident.

- When buying electric tools for use in the garden, for greater safety, select those which are double-insulated.
- Some electric mowers are designed to stop within a few seconds of being switched off, while others have blades that continue to rotate momentarily after being switched off. If you can, choose the former because, in an accident, the quicker the blades come to a standstill, the better.
- Never join two power cables to make a longer one or repair a cut by making a join. Taped joins pull apart and aren't waterproof. Buy a new cable.
- Ensure all exterior cables are bright orange or yellow, so they stand out against the green of your lawn.
- Switch off and unplug a mower, edge trimmer or bandsaw before you attempt to unclog it, or do any other work on it, such as lubricating, cleaning or adjusting.
- If you are up a ladder when using a hedge trimmer, work only within comfortable arm's reach. Rather climb down and move the ladder than risk a fall by stretching too far.
- Always use a chain saw as directed. The chain rotates away from you on the top pass, and towards you along the lower cutting edge so that if it jumps or jams, it will jump away from you rather than towards you. Never try to cut using the top pass of the chain.
- When mowing the lawn, wear shoes that cover your feet completely, with soles that minimize the risk of slipping.
- Use eye protection, as clippings and flying debris could be driven into your eyes.
- Never use an electric mower in the early morning when there is still dew present, in the rain or just after rain has fallen.

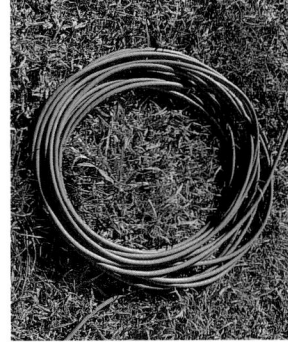

Brightly coloured extension cables stand out against the grass.

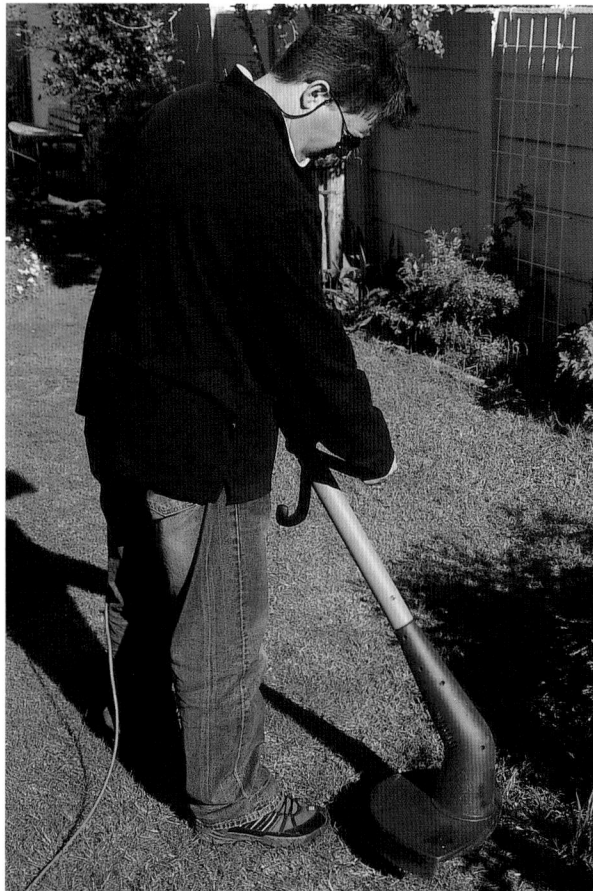

The power cable should always be behind you.

- Always work away from the cable to minimize the risk of cutting it.
- Always use a cable with a rating that is correct for the machine, or greater. Using too thin a cable could lead to it becoming overheated.
- Never bypass the safety switch on an electric tool. The switch is designed to stop the tool when it is released (for instance, if you slip).
- When checking the cutting parts of a petrol mower, switch it off and pull off the spark plug lead before turning the machine on its side. If you fail to take this precaution and turn the blades by hand, to remove grass clippings for example, the engine may start, and even one or two revolutions can result in severe injury.

- Always push a mower, never pull it, except perhaps to remove it from a confined area, such as between two flower beds. On longer runs, push – if you slip while pulling it towards you, your feet or hands could be injured.
- Work across slopes, not straight down or up; if you slip while pushing up a slope, the mower might roll down on you; if you slip down onto the mower, your feet could be injured.

STORING GARDEN TOOLS

- A safe and effective way to store large garden implements such as forks and spades is to place them 'sharp end' down in a big bin.
- Alternatively, attach a length of timber to the wall with two shorter lengths so that the beam stands clear by 15cm (6in) or so. Stack long-handled garden tools behind it. The front surface can be used to hang smaller items, such as potting trowels or secateurs.

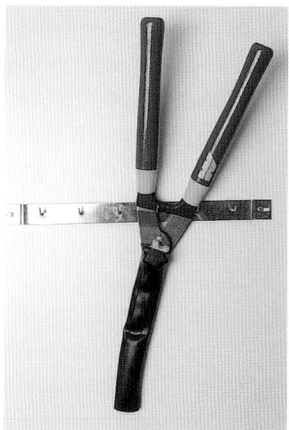

- Keep the blades of garden shears closed by slipping a length of bicycle inner tube over the ends. This prevents the points from doing any real harm if the shears fall on anyone.
- If you need to store a pitchfork or three-pronged fork with the prongs uppermost, slip lengths of old garden hose over each tine to stop the points injuring anyone.

Cover the blades of unused garden shears with rubber tubing and store facing down.

- Never leave a rake lying on the ground with its prongs up – the experience of stepping on one and having the handle fly up into your face is something you won't forget in a hurry.

Reducing natural plant dangers

Even the best-tended garden can be a dangerous trap for the unwary. Different plants pose differing degrees of danger, from downright deadly to reasonably benign. While most of us would consider ourselves safe in our own gardens, we can get scratched by branches, prick ourselves on thorns or get sap or pollen in our eyes. Unless you are certain of your identification, it is best to assume that any unknown plant poses a risk, even if it is just of an irritating rash. On a more serious level though, while adults don't normally go around putting bits of plants into their mouths, children certainly do, and if a curious child 'investigates' poisonous leaves, berries or fruits, it is easy to have a poisoning emergency on your hands.

Every region and climate is home to common garden plants you need to watch out for. Some are widespread, others are endemic to a small area. Get to know the local plants of your region, and ask your garden centre or nursery for advice before selecting unfamiliar plants, particularly if you have toddlers or pets in the home. Some flowers and trees produce copious amounts of pollen, or have fine fibres or spores that can irritate the airway of individuals susceptible to allergies or asthma. If you are affected, getting rid of the offending plants is probably the only solution.

Many attractive garden plants are poisonous. Sometimes the whole plant is deadly, but often only one part of the plant is affected, perhaps the berries, roots, bulbs or leaves; the sap of oleander bushes for example, can cause painful inflammation if it enters the eyes. The thorns of the firethorn (*Pyracantha*) can cause blisters if the point penetrates the skin. Some plants are poisonous in their raw state but, when properly prepared, become part of dinner. Rhubarb is a good example: the leaves should not be consumed or fed to pets, but the edible stems are delicious when cooked.

Plants with thorns or spines pose a special danger. Although they may have a specific function, such as to create a secure border or hedge, they are often integrated with normal plantings. While everybody knows to keep clear of cacti or rose bushes, many plants and weeds have tiny spines or thorns that are less visible, but which can inflict a nasty scratch, sting or puncture, as experienced by anyone who has had a close encounter with stinging nettles (*Urtica dioica*).

When considering whether to plant thorny species, bear in mind their placement within the garden. A sisal plant (*Agave sisalana*), its fleshy leaves edged with thorns and tipped with a formidable spike, poses a danger at the best of times, but if it is located at the bottom of a grassy bank where children roll and play, the implications are magnified.

When it comes to safety, the best rule of thumb for gardeners is to know which plants are dangerous and where they are located, and make sure that everyone in the family, including children, is aware of them and why they should leave them alone. Ultimately if, despite doing everything you can to teach your children what not to do, you are still concerned, removing the offending plants is probably the safest route to take.

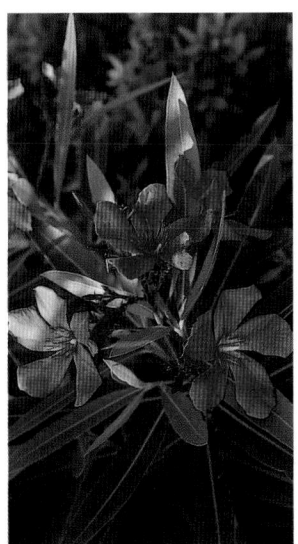

The oleander is very poisonous.

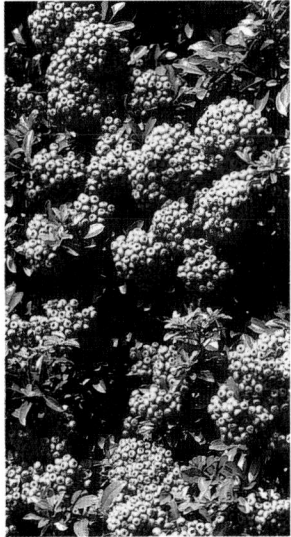

Firethorn can cause painful blisters.

WATER SAFETY

In warm climates, recreation in and on water is high on the list of preferred pastimes. When the sun is hot, we enjoy spending days at the beach, frolicking by the river or lazing around the pool. But, while many people think only in terms of swimming when it comes to safety and responsible behaviour in water, pastimes such as boating, fishing or scuba diving, also demand proper attention to safety, particularly when they take place at sea, where weather and tidal conditions come into play. Whenever you venture onto the water, pay attention to local weather and water conditions. Get out of, or off, the water at the first sign of approaching bad weather, particularly if it looks like a storm accompanied by lightning. As much as water gives us pleasure, failing to treat it with respect can prove fatal. Parents of toddlers need to be especially vigilant and maintain constant supervision anywhere near water, as drowning can occur in only a few centimetres of water. Although we consider young children to be most at risk, anyone, regardless of age, can get into trouble if basic common-sense and safety precautions are not followed in and around water.

IN THIS SECTION

Basic rules around water

SWIMMERS

- Learn to swim. Children can begin swimming lessons from a young age. If you have a pool at home, it is worth teaching your child to swim, and to respect water, as early as possible.
- Never swim alone, even in your own pool, as you never know when you might get into difficulties. At the beach or lake, swim only in areas protected by lifeguards.
- Obey all rules and posted signs regarding swimming, boating and water sports.
- Watch out for the 'dangerous too's'– too tired, too cold, too far from safety, too much sun, too much strenuous activity.
- Remember that swim aids, flotation devices and inflatable pool toys cannot replace parental supervision. Swim aids can suddenly slip or shift out of position, or an inflatable toy could lose air, leaving the child in a dangerous situation.

- Don't mix alcohol and water. Alcohol impairs your judgement, balance and coordination, affects your swimming, diving skills and motor coordination, and reduces your body's ability to stay warm.

BOATERS

- Ensure that you are familiar with the rules and regulations governing the use of powered craft, including jet skis, and obey them. Don't go boating in restricted waters, or operate your craft recklessly, or if you are under the influence of alcohol – the penalties are likely to be severe. Furthermore, if anyone is injured as a result of your negligent behaviour you may face civil action.

Water games are fun, but even the most innocent paddle in a baby pool can turn into a disaster. Be alert and on the lookout for trouble and don't rely on others to look after your child.

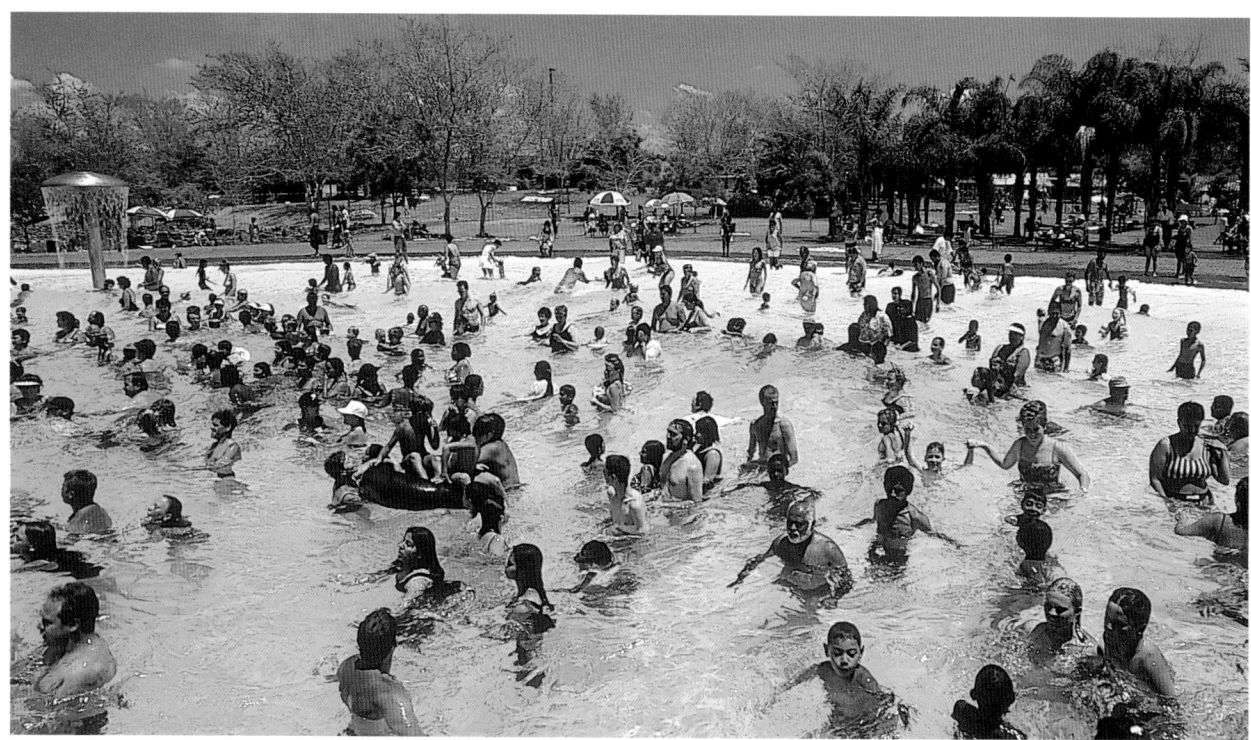

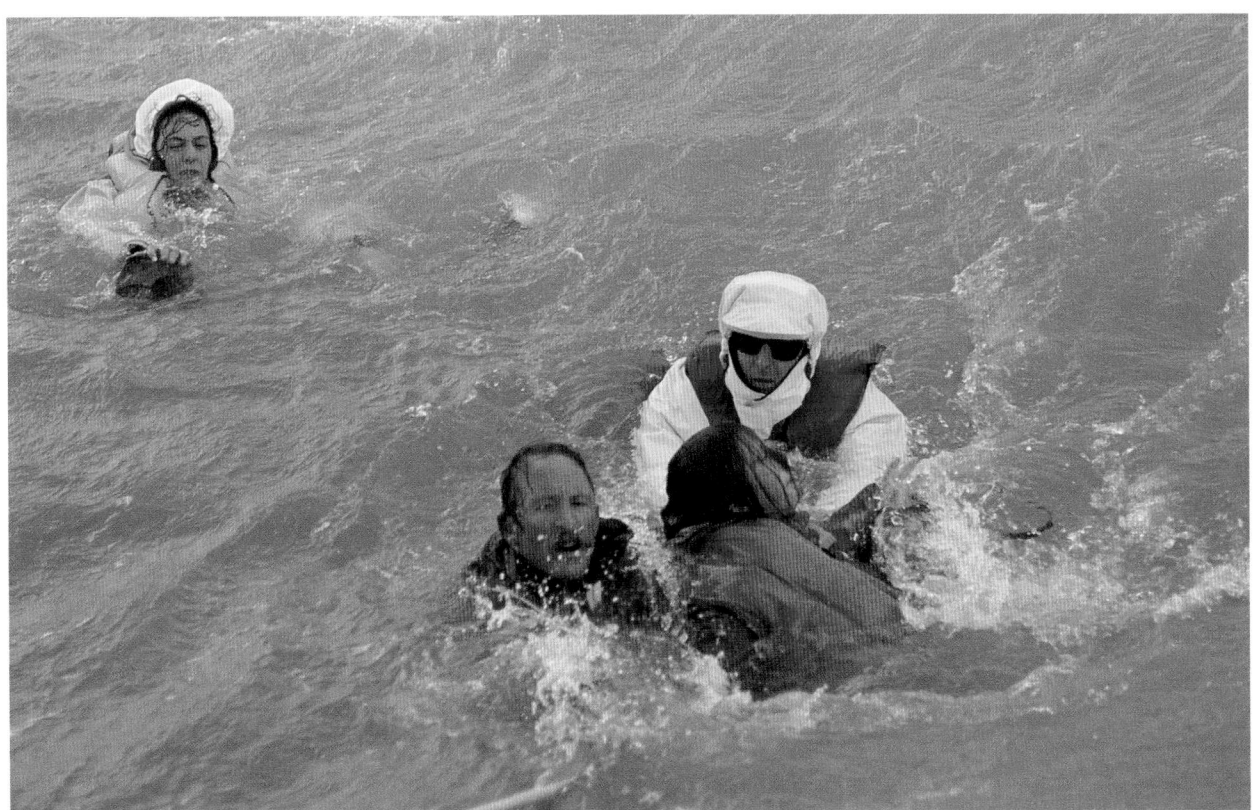

A professional rescue operation in progress.

LEGAL ASPECTS

When it comes to issues of safety, the law is usually on the side of the victim. 'What would a reasonable person be reasonably expected to think' is a question to bear in mind when considering circumstances that might cause injury, particularly if they occur as a result of negligence. Every case is different, but if you fail to take reasonable precautions with regard to the possible impact on the safety and wellbeing of others, you could be faced with criminal and/or civil actions of immense gravity. Ignorance of the law is no excuse, though it might affect whether an accused is deemed to have intended to commit the crime or not (in legal terminology this is called mens rea). But don't count on it.

THE IMPLICATIONS OF BEING RESCUED

The cost of rescuing a swimmer, sailor or anyone else in trouble on the water can be considerable. While the lifeguard who dives in and brings you to shore with little more than wounded pride may

expect nothing more than a heartfelt 'thank you' and perhaps a donation to a rescue organization, in some countries, the cost of a rescue can be considerable. Rescue services are not always paid for by the state and you may be presented with a large bill, particularly if your own negligence or stupidity was the cause of the incident.

If you defy warnings and swim when conditions are hazardous and then get into difficulties, you could be held responsible for the cost of any operation required to rescue you, and face legal action for putting the lives of your rescuers at risk. Likewise, putting to sea in a small boat when a storm is approaching is foolhardy and the cost of effecting a rescue could be substantial.

Coastguard or private rescue craft, helicopters and emergency medical services all cost money to operate; if it is deemed that you are responsible for your predicament, you will have to reimburse the costs. If you spend a lot of time on the water, in whatever capacity, ask your insurance broker to amend your policy to cover any rescue services you may require.

Children and water

It is a sad global statistic that most drownings of children under the age of four occur in home swimming pools. By strictly adhering to the safety regulations and ensuring that you pay undivided attention when your youngsters are splashing around in or near the water on a hot summer's day you will be able to prevent tragedy. City and local bylaws and ordinances vary from place to place and may change from time to time. If you intend building a pool or pond, make sure that you are familiar with what is required in terms of perimeter fencing, gates and other safety devices and precautions. Although most reputable contractors will be able to advise you, remember that the onus is on you to inform yourself and then to comply. Failure to do so could lead to civil or criminal action being taken against you in the event of an accident.

PONDS AND SWIMMING POOLS

While ponds or swimming pools are undoubtedly an asset that enhances a property's value and provides a lot of enjoyment, they claim lives every year, so never leave a child unobserved anywhere near water. Adult supervision is recommended at all times when children are around water.

- Restrict access to the water by enclosing it with a secure fence and a self-locking, self-closing gate. The fence should have vertical bars with openings no more than 10cm (4in) wide. Keep the gate locked when a pool is not being used. Any doors leading directly from the house to the area should also remain locked. Add further protection with an alarm or sensor system that makes a loud noise when the gate is opened.
- A resourceful child may find a way to climb over a fence, so be careful where you leave garden furniture or other items that can be easily moved to provide a handy step.

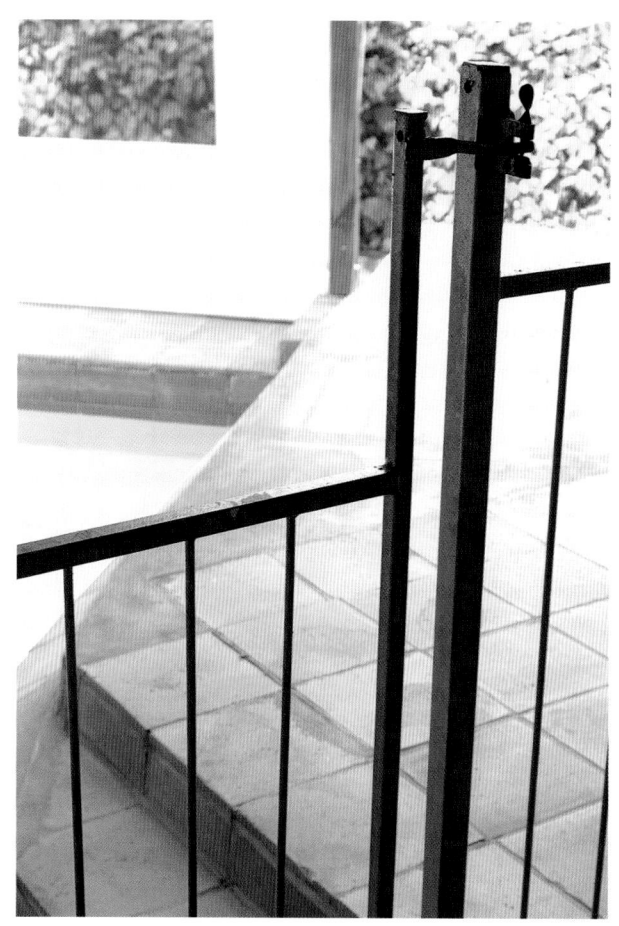

Enclose your swimming pool with a sturdy fence and ensure the gate is kept securely locked, especially when you are not around.

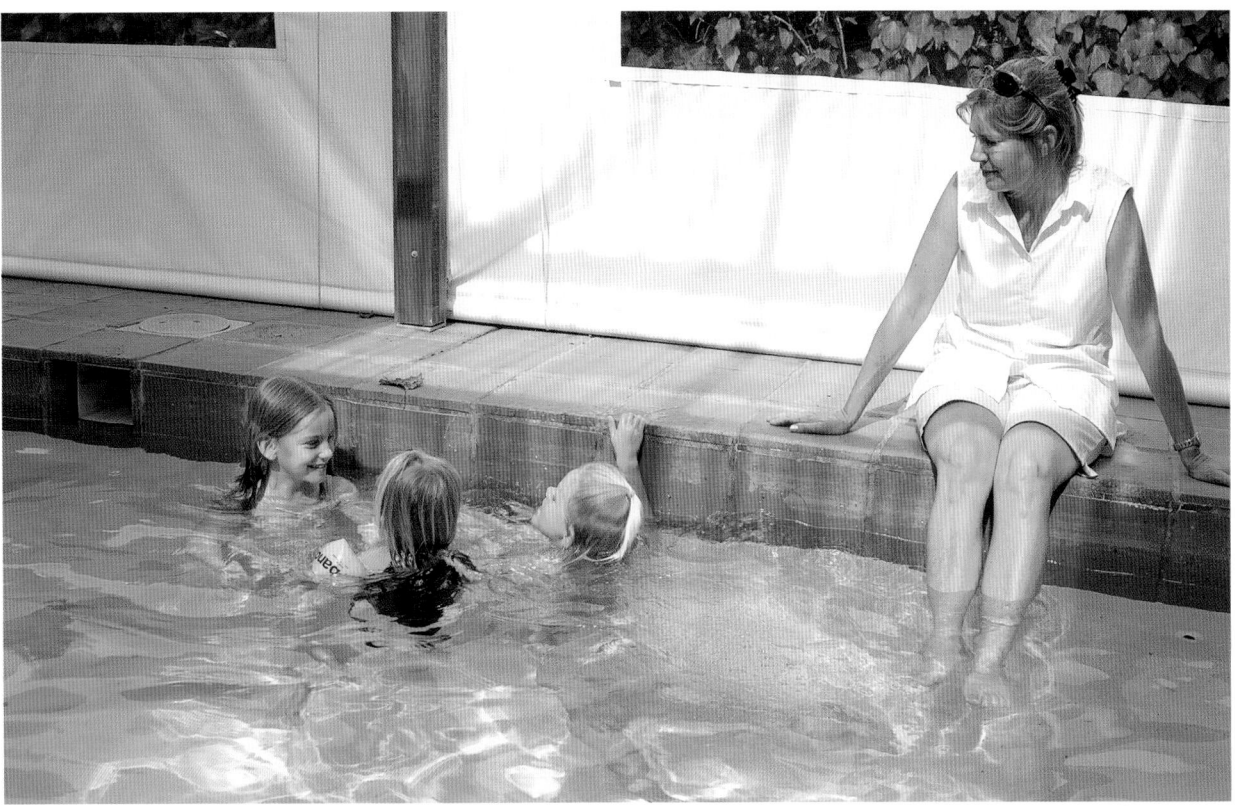

Always make sure that a competent adult is present when children are in the swimming pool.

- Keep basic lifesaving equipment near the pool. A sturdy pole, length of nylon rope and flotation devices are recommended.
- Toys can attract young children into the pool area, so pack them away after use. Floating toys are particularly dangerous as children may fall into the water while trying to retrieve them.
- Water makes some pool surrounds very slippery, so teach your children not to run around the pool. They should also not jump or dive in without checking first to see whether there is someone else on the surface or under the water.
- If a child goes missing in the home, check the pool area first. Go to the edge of the pool and scan the entire pool, bottom and surface, as well as the surrounding area. Hide-and-seek is a great game, but not around a pool.
- Buoyancy devices (swim aids) must have safety approval and must be appropriate for the age of the child. A small child is more top-heavy than an adult; if the design is faulty or the fit is wrong, the child could end up floating face-down.

- Swimming pool parties increase the risk of accidents. Ensure there are sufficient adult supervisors present, focus your attention on the children and keep a mobile (cellular) or cordless phone nearby so that you can call for assistance in an emergency.
- Learn **rescue breathing** (*see* p26) and **resuscitation** (*see* pp22–37) and insist that your children's properly trained. Display resuscitation instructions somewhere close to the pool area, and keep a list of your local emergency response numbers near the telephone.

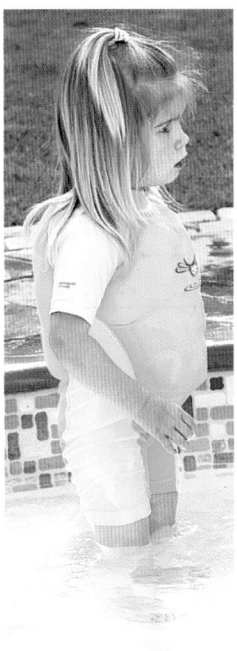

Swim aids must fit well in order to be effective.

- Store pool chemicals securely. Chlorine, pool acid and other chemicals are hazardous if mishandled and you don't want your budding scientist conducting experiments to see what might happen when they mix. The result could be severe burns, even the loss of a hand or eye.
- Make sure your pool's pump system is covered and that the power cable leading to it is buried underground and well protected from inadvertent damage by a garden fork. Ideally, sheath the cable in a conduit to protect the insulation and bury it at a depth of at least 30cm (12in). You can reinforce the safety aspect if you place bricks or paving slabs on top of the conduit before refilling the trench. For future reference, make a note of the position of the cable on your house plans, including a note stating how deep it has been buried and how it is protected.

PONDS AND WATER FEATURES

Virtually any body of water is appealing to toddlers and young children but, as they are naturally inquisitive and resourceful, in order to keep them safe, you must ensure that even the most remote chance of an accident is neutralized.

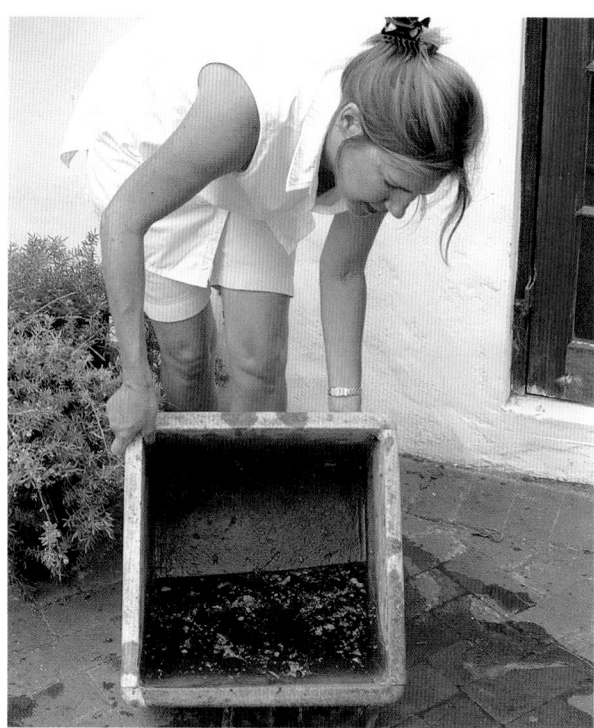

Empty rain-filled plant pots that are not in use.

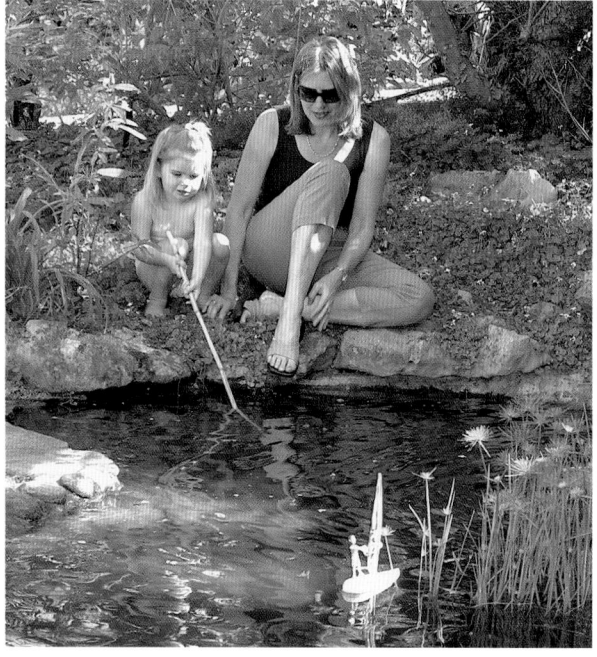

- If power is required, select a pump that operates at a lower voltage than your normal mains current. In such a case, the step-down transformer will be close to the mains plug-in point, with the low-voltage cable (buried and protected as with a pool cable) going into the garden and to the pump. Electricity and water don't usually mix, nor does electricity and a garden fork, so check with your local authority beforehand to ensure that you abide by the regulations when laying the cable to the pond. When working on a pool or pond pump, switch off the power and unplug the connection before doing the job.
- If you have an external rain butt or water collection tank, make sure that the lid is securely padlocked at all times. After heavy rains, make a habit of emptying buckets, plant pots or other garden containers into which a toddler could fall.

Always make sure to have an adult nearby when children are playing around a water feature.

Public waters

It is impossible to cover all aspects of safety on public waters. There are too many individual variables to take into account, not least of which is our own attitude towards safety and the behaviour and attitude of those with whom share the water. All the basic rules of water safety apply when you are swimming or boating on public waterways, but perhaps the most important one is never to get into unfamiliar water without taking the time to consider the potential dangers and assess the risks. Many local authorities demarcate specific areas for swimming, non-motorized water sports (such as surfing and sail boarding) and boating, but if there are no notices to this effect, you might find boats being launched in areas where swimmers, surfers and sailboarders play, so pick your beach or water frontage carefully. Despite regulations governing access to open water there are often grey areas when it comes to small craft. It goes without saying that responsible boat-owners comply with the relevant statutory requirements and are properly qualified to operate a vessel before they take to the water. If you take your sail-boat, powerboat or jet ski on holiday with you, ensure you observe the local rules, are familiar with the conditions, and have the local emergency numbers close at hand.

SAFETY AT SEA AND IN RIVERS

- Check surf and water conditions. If there are warning flags up (these vary from country to country), observe them.
- Select a supervised area. A lifeguard who can help in an emergency is the best safety factor.
- Even good swimmers can have an unexpected emergency in the water, so never swim alone.
- If there are no supervised areas, select a spot that has good water quality and safe conditions. Murky or churning water, hidden rocks, unexpected drop-offs, and aquatic plants are hazards. Strong tides, currents and big waves can spell tragedy. In rivers and lakes, water pollution can cause health problems for swimmers.
- Never jump or dive into water unless you are positive of its depth. Every year, many swimmers suffer serious neck and spinal cord injuries from diving headfirst into water that is too shallow.

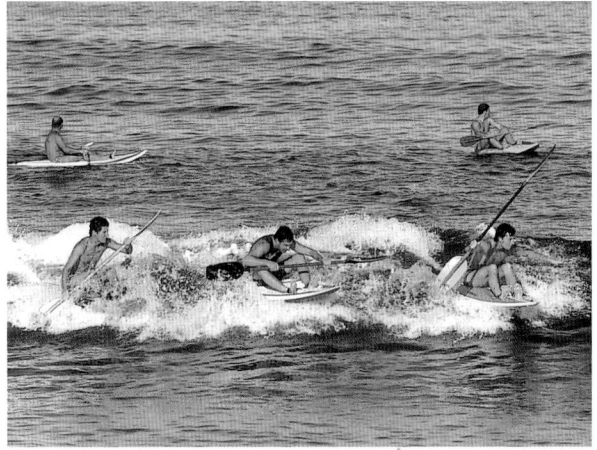

The sea is unpredictable so always be alert.

Remember that tides and wave movement can alter the depth of the water and create sand bars where there were none before.

- Don't swim too far from the shore, or too far up- or downriver, and make sure you always have enough energy to swim back, particularly if it is against a current. If you get caught in a crosscurrent, don't try to swim against it. Swim gradually out of the current by swimming across it.
- Be sure that docks and floating rafts are in good condition. A well-run open-water facility maintains its rafts and docks in good condition, with no loose boards or exposed nails. Never swim under a raft or dock. Always look before jumping off a dock or raft to be sure no one is in the way. When in the sea, stay away from piers, pilings, mooring buoys and scuba diving platforms.
- If you get caught in river rapids, keep your legs together, arms outspread and face downstream so that you can spot rocks or overhanging branches ahead and avoid them. Don't try to stand up. Rather crawl over to the nearest shore, cutting across the current. If you swim against it, you are unlikely to get anywhere very quickly.
- In lakes and rivers, drainage ditches built to handle water run-off are dangerous. After heavy rains, they can quickly change into raging rivers that can easily take a human life. Debris picked up by the rushing water adds to the danger.

- On rivers, a sharp bend tends to shelve towards the outer edge of the bend where the water is deepest and the bank is often steep and under-cut. A swiftly flowing current will push you towards this deeper, outer area and you could be out of your depth very quickly.
- Whether you are going to the beach or to the shore of a lake or river, select an area that is well maintained. Clean restrooms and a litter-free environment show the management's concern for your health and safety.

BOATING AND MOTORIZED WATER ACTIVITIES

- Sign up for one of the many recognized training courses that are available. These will teach you general water safety and rescue techniques and prepare you for all eventualities.
- Before taking your boat out, sign out at the club, or give a responsible person details about the direction you plan to go in and how long you expect to be gone. If you do not have radio or cell-phone contact, do not deviate from your plan – certainly not substantially anyway. This is important because if you are delayed by a change in the weather, become lost, or encounter any other problems, you want help to be able to reach you.

In rivers, follow the current feet first so that you can see obstacles in your path.

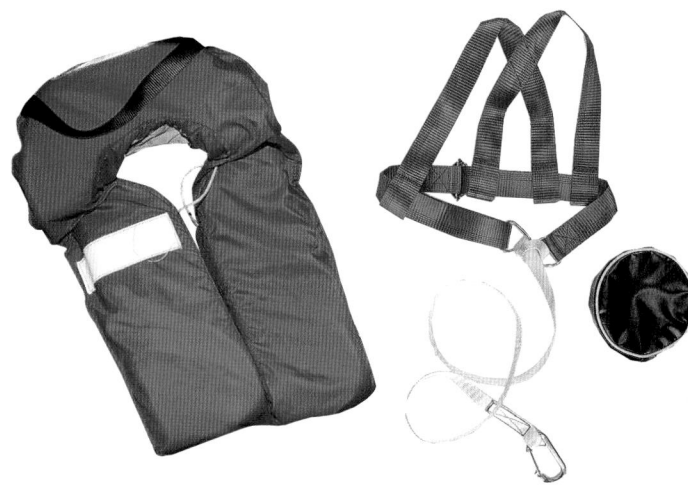

A life jacket and a harness must be worn at all times when boating or fishing.

- Approved life jackets or safety harnesses must be worn at all times, even when fishing. Children's jackets should be correct for body size and weight.
- Keep a watch for vessels or activities on and in the water. Be aware of boats that may have divers or snorkellers in the water, and of boardsailors trying to right their craft. Slow down when passing, and clear the area by a wide margin.
- Operate your craft with courtesy and common sense. Follow the traffic pattern of the waterway, keep to marked channels and adhere to the 'rules of the road' as indicated by navigation buoys and/or lights. Obey no-wake and maximum speed zones, and watch the water ahead of you at all times. Do not operate the boat at night or in restricted areas.
- Power boat operators should use extreme caution around swimmers and surfers. Maintain a slow speed until your craft is away from the shore, swimming areas and docks. Avoid passing too close to other boats, or jumping wakes.

The rules of the 'road' state that sail must give way to larger, powered vessels in a narrow channel.

- Jet skiers should always travel in groups of two or more as you never know when an emergency might occur. When you are far from shore, even running out of petrol constitutes an emergency, particularly if the wind is blowing you out to sea!
- Ensure your equipment is in good shape and operating properly before setting off.
- When water-skiing, boat operators must turn the motor off when approaching a fallen skier. Have a person aboard to watch and assist the skier, who should use proper hand signals to communicate with the boat operator. When coming in to land, skiers should run parallel to the shore and come in slowly. Sit down if you are coming in too fast.
- Alcohol and boats don't mix for the same reasons as drinking and driving (impaired judgement, lack of concentration and a greater propensity for accidents), so keep these activities separate.

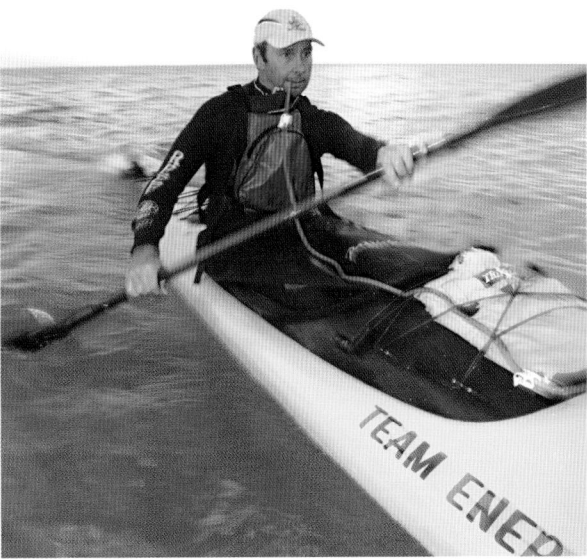

If you are planning a longer kayaking trip, ensure that you are suitably equipped.

NON-MOTORIZED WATERCRAFT

- Never go out alone. If you are new to an area, watch the locals and ask questions about the wind and wave conditions before putting to sea.
- Board sailors must always wear an approved life jacket or safety harness and check all their equipment before setting out.
- For rafting or tubing on white water a buoyancy aid, PFD and protective helmet are essential.
- In cold conditions, surfers and board sailors should wear a full wetsuit to prevent hypothermia. On sunny days, a long top and sun-block (sunscreen) will help to reduce the risk of wind- and sunburn.

Personal flotation device (PFD)

- Remember that you need good physical strength and swimming ability for most water sports. Being on a board or tube does not negate the need to be able to swim!
- Do not overload a raft or tube.
- Watch out for swimmers and other water users, particularly when coming around a bend in a river.
- Do not go rafting or boating in rivers after a heavy downpour, as flash floods may occur.

SNORKELLING AND SCUBA DIVING

- If you are new to snorkelling, practise in shallow water until you feel confident. Check your equipment carefully and know how it functions. Learn how to clear water from the snorkel and how to put your mask back on while you tread water.
- Be careful not to swim or be carried by a current too far from shore or the boat.
- Observe the 'buddy' rule and never dive alone or snorkel alone in deep waters.
- No reputable dive operator will sell, hire or refill a scuba cylinder unless you produce a valid C-card (diving licence), so there are no short-cuts to proper lessons and certification before venturing underwater. Once certified, do not dive in environments for which you are not qualified. Your dive master or boat operator should ensure that you are trained and equipped for any dive you are about to undertake.
- Responsible divers 'plan the dive and dive the plan'. When underwater, do not deviate from your agreed plan. Monitor your underwater time and remaining air, allowing for any decompression stops you may have to make on the way up.
- A common mistake novice scuba divers make is to dive when they have a cold, sinus infection or other respiratory ailment. You will not be able to equalize properly, resulting in a painful and unpleasant dive.

WATER THEME-PARKS

- Be sure the area is supervised by lifeguards. Read all posted signs, follow any directions given by the lifeguards and ask questions if you are not sure about the correct procedure.
- When you go from one attraction to another, remember that the water depth may differ.
- Before you start down a water slide, get into the correct position – face up and feet first.
- Some facilities provide life jackets at no charge. Anyone who cannot swim should wear a life jacket on all rides and attractions.

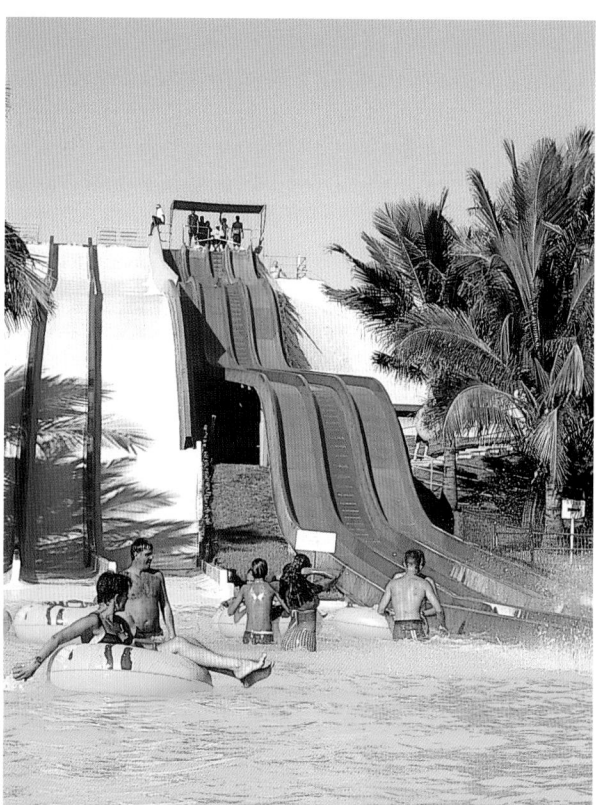

Safe diving means making sure that your equipment is in good working order before you enter the water.

Keep a careful eye on your child at all times in a water theme-park. It could slip and fall, or be pushed into deep water – so be alert.

BASIC LIFESAVING TIPS

RESCUING YOURSELF

If you find yourself in trouble, there are steps you can take to help yourself while you wait to be rescued.

- As you fall in, hold your breath and close your mouth to avoid swallowing water. Once in the water, try to stand – some rivers and dams may not be as deep as they seem.
- If you cannot stand, and the shore is some distance away, tread water. Keep your body upright and use your hands and feet to 'pedal' towards the shore or nearest safe object.
- If you are wearing heavy or bulky clothing or shoes, see if you can remove them, and perhaps even use them as flotation devices.
- Reduce the loss of body heat by adopting a sitting position in the water, drawing your knees up and hugging them to your chest.
- If you can swim, and conditions allow it, make for the nearest shore. Go with the flow of the current and swim with a stroke that does not tire you too quickly, especially if you have some distance to cover. If you get tired, float on your back or tread water for a while.
- If someone throws you a life ring or some form of flotation device, make sure you get a firm grasp on it, so that they can tow you to shore. If the current is strong, or there are breaking waves, try to use the natural ebb and flow to assist the rescuer, but allow them to take control of the situation.

HELPING OTHERS

- Do not attempt to rescue someone else unless you have had training and know what to do.
- If you need to rescue someone else from deep water, be aware that they are likely to panic, and could force you underwater.
- Do not swim out unless there is no other means of reaching the person. Take something they can hold onto, such as a life ring, or rescue buoy. Improvise with a towel or piece of clothing if there is nothing else to hand.

MOUTH-TO-MOUTH RESUSCITATION

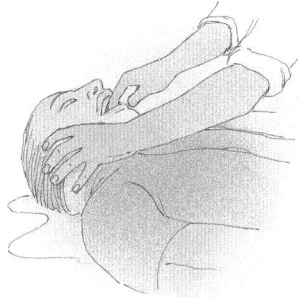

1. *Gently tilt the head back and lift the chin to open the airway. Ensure that nothing restricts breathing.*

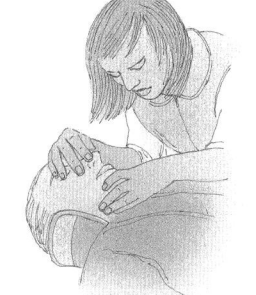

2. *Pinch the nostrils closed, take a deep breath, place your mouth firmly over his.*

3. *Exhale deeply into his mouth for two seconds and see if the chest rises. If it doesn't check the airway for blockage.*

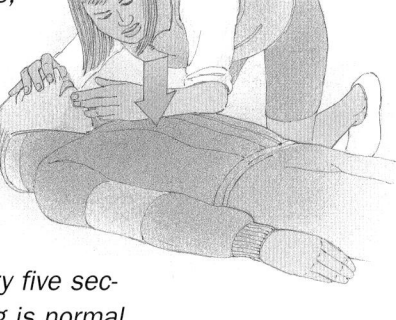

4. *As his chest falls, breathe in again deeply and repeat. Check the pulse to see if the heart is beating. If it is, continue breathing into his mouth every five seconds until breathing is normal. Then place in the recovery position.*

QUICK REMINDER – SAFE

In an emergency, the last thing you need is to wonder 'what should I do next?' By memorizing the well-tested sequence of actions summarized below and on the opposite page, you will be able to take effective action in those first vital minutes of an emergency situation.

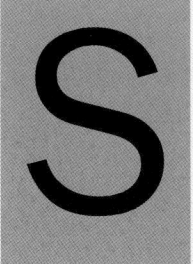

SHOUT FOR HELP
Summon medical assistance or the emergency services immediately. The ideal is to send a responsible person to make the call while you immediately begin attending to the casualty.

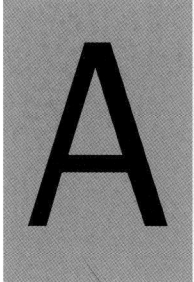

APPROACH WITH CARE
Check the surroundings for any hazard that might endanger you or the casualty. This also includes an assessment of the casualty's state of mind.

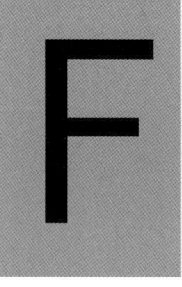

FREE FROM DANGER
Even though a casualty should not be moved until the emergency services arrive, this must be weighed against any further risk to the casualty or to yourself and any other rescuers.

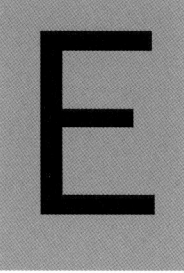

EVALUATE THE ABC
Having taken the above precautions, you are now ready to assess the level of consciousness and the casualty's vital functions (the ABC) and commence resuscitation if required.

QUICK REMINDER – ABC

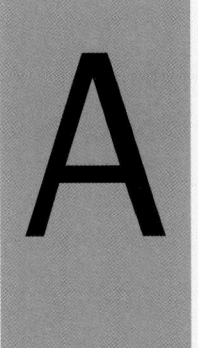

AIRWAY
An unconscious person may need to have his airway cleared to enable him to breathe on his own. Turn the casualty onto his back and use head tilt and chin lift to position the head (*see* p24). If a neck injury is suspected, support the head carefully during any movement; first try the chin lift alone.

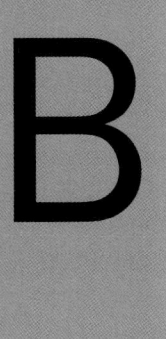

BREATHING
Having positioned and cleared the airway, you need to establish whether the casualty is breathing, by looking for chest movement, listening for sounds of breathing, and feeling for exhaled breath. If there are no signs of breathing within 10 seconds, give rescue breaths (*see* p24).

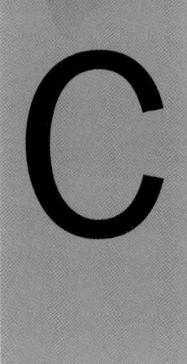

CIRCULATION
If the casualty is breathing, or has resumed breathing once the airway is cleared, check the circulation by feeling for a pulse in the carotid artery (below the jawbone) or brachial artery (at the elbow joint). If you cannot feel a pulse within 10 seconds, start chest compressions (*see* p26).

GLOSSARY

A

ABC Acronym meaning A = Airway; B = Breathing; C = Circulation.

Abdominal thrust The manual thrusts to create a pressure wave to expel an airway obstruction.

Abrasion A scraped or scratched skin wound.

Acute A condition that comes on quickly and has severe symptoms (*see* **chronic** for comparison).

Airway The route for air into and out of the lungs.

Allergens Substances which trigger an allergic reaction in the body.

Amputation Complete removal of a body part.

Anaphylaxis An exaggerated allergic reaction; may be rapidly fatal.

Angina (pectoris) Sudden pain in the chest due to a lack of blood supply to the heart muscle.

Arteries Blood vessels that carry blood away from the heart (see also Veins).

Arteriosclerosis A name for several conditions that cause the walls of the arteries to become thick, hard and inelastic.

Asthma Attacks of difficult breathing with wheezing and/or coughing, often due to allergens.

Atherosclerosis A form of arteriosclerosis caused by fat deposits in the arterial walls.

B

Back blows Sharp blows to the upper back, done to relieve an airway obstruction.

Bacteria Germs which can cause disease.

Basic life support Maintaining the ABCs without equipment.

Blood pressure The pressure of blood against the walls of arterial blood vessels.

Blood volume The total amount of blood in the heart and blood vessels.

Brachial pulse Pulse felt on the inner upper arm, usually taken on infants.

Bruise Broken blood vessels under the skin.

C

Capillaries Very small blood vessels that link the arteries and the veins and allow gases and nutrients to move into and out of the tissues.

Capillary refill test A test to determine whether a person is in shock: press on the casualty's finger tip for five seconds and then release. If the normal pink skin colour does not return within two seconds, the person suffers from **shock** (*see* p38).

Carbon dioxide (CO_2) A waste gas produced by the cells and breathed out via the lungs.

Carbon monoxide (CO) A dangerous, colourless and odourless gas which displaces the carrying of oxygen by the red blood cells.

Cardiovascular disease Refers to disorders of the heart and blood vessels, such as high blood pressure and arteriosclerosis.

Cardiac arrest The sudden stopping of cardiac function with no pulse, and unresponsiveness.

Carotid artery The main artery of the neck, used to assess the carotid pulse.

Cartilage A tough, rubbery tissue that covers the surfaces where bones meet, and also forms part of the nose and ears.

Central nervous system Part of the nervous system consisting of the brain and the spinal cord.

Cerebrovascular accident (CVA) A stroke, or the sudden stopping of circulation to part of the brain.

Cervical collar A device used to immobilize and support the neck.

Chest thrusts Series of manual thrusts to the chest to relieve airway obstruction in infants and children.

Cholesterol A fatty substance found in animal tissue or products, also produced by the body. It is thought to contribute to arteriosclerosis.

Chronic A long-standing, persistent or relapsing condition or illness.

Chronic obstructive pulmonary disease (COPD) A term describing a group of chronic lung diseases that cause obstructions in the airway and lungs.

Circulatory system The heart and blood vessels.

Closed wound Where the skin is intact.

Concussion A temporary disturbance of brain function, usually caused by a blow to the head.

Congestive heart failure Failure of the heart to pump effectively, causing a back up of fluid in the lungs and body tissues.

Coronary artery Vessel which feeds the heart muscle.

Cornea The transparent front part of the eyeball.

Croup A group of viral infections that cause swelling of the inner throat, particularly in infants and children.

Cyanosis A bluish or grey colour of the skin due to insufficient oxygen in the blood, or poor circulation.

D

Defibrillation Applying an electrical shock to a fibrillating heart (see Fibrillation).

Deoxygenated blood Blood containing a low level of oxygen.

Diabetes A disease caused by lack of insulin, or insulin resistance, which causes excess blood sugar.

Diarrhoea Frequent soft or watery bowel movements.

Direct pressure Force applied directly to a wound to help stop bleeding.

Dislocation When bone surfaces at a joint are out of alignment.

Dressing A covering over a wound, used to stop bleeding and prevent contamination.

E

Embedded object A foreign object stuck in the skin or impaled in body tissue.

Embolus Any foreign matter, such as a blood clot, fat clump or air bubble carried in the blood stream.

Emetic A substance which causes vomiting.

EMS Emergency Medical Services system; a community's group of services which respond to emergencies.

Emphysema A chronic lung disease characterized by overstretched alveolar walls (see COPD).

Epidermis The outer-most layer of skin.

Epiglottis A lid-like piece of tissue which protects the entrance to the larynx (voice-box).

Epiglottitis Infection, usually in children, resulting in a swelling of the epiglottis (may cause croup).

Epilepsy A chronic brain disorder characterized by recurrent convulsions.

ESM Emergency Scene Management – the sequence of actions a first aider should follow to give safe and appropriate first aid.

Exhalation Expiration, or breathing out.

F

Fibrillation Uncoordinated ineffective contractions of the heart muscle.

Flail chest A condition in which several ribs are broken in at least two places, creating a segment that does not move normally.

First aid The help given to an injured or suddenly ill person, using readily available materials.

First aider Someone who takes charge of an emergency scene and gives first aid.

First responders People such as the police, fire fighters, ambulance attendants, etc. who are called first to an emergency scene.

Fontanelle The soft gaps between the bones of the skull that can be felt on babies' heads.

Fracture A cracked or broken bone.

Frostbite Tissue damage as a result of exposure to extremely cold conditions.

G

Gastric distention A swelling of the stomach, usually with air, due to ventilating with excessive volume or force during artificial respiration.

Gauze An open mesh material used for dressings.

Glasgow Coma Scale (modified) A method of estimating the casualty's level of consciousness.

H

Head-tilt chin-lift manoeuvre Opening the casualty's airway by tilting the head backward and lifting the chin forward.

Heart attack Chest pain due to a death of a part of the heart muscle; a myocardial infarction.

Heart failure A weakened heart muscle that is unable to push blood forward; fluid backs up into the lungs, causing swelling of the ankles etc.

Heat cramps Painful muscle spasms due to excessive loss of fluid and salts by sweating.

Heat stroke A life-threatening emergency where the temperature regulation mechanism cannot cool the body and the temperature is far above normal; also called hyperthermia or sunstroke.

Heimlich manoeuvre (*see* **abdominal thrusts**).

History Information about the casualty's problem, symptoms, events leading up to the problem, applicable illnesses or medications, etc.

Hyperglycaemia Abnormally high blood sugar.

Hypertension High blood pressure.

Hyperthermia Too high body temperature.

Hyperventilation Too deep or rapid respirations.

Hypoglycaemia Too low blood sugar levels.

Hypothermia Too low body temperature.

Hypoxia Too low levels of oxygen in the tissues.

I

Impaled object Object embedded in a wound.

Immobilization Placing some type of restraint along a body part to prevent movement.

Incontinence Loss of bladder or bowel control.

Infarction An area of tissue death due to lack of blood flow.

Inflammation A tissue reaction to irritation, illness or injury; shows as redness, heat, swelling or pain.

Inhalation Breathing in, inspiration.

Insulin Hormone produced by the pancreas; important in the regulation of blood sugar levels.

Insulin coma/shock Too low blood sugar levels (hypoglycaemia) due to excessive insulin.

Involuntary muscle Muscles not under conscious control, such as the heart, intestines etc.

Ischaemic Lacking sufficient oxygen; as in ischaemic heart disease.

J

Joint A place where two or more bones meet.

Joint capsule A tough covering over a joint.

L

Laceration A jagged wound from a rip or tear.

Ligament A tough cord of tissue which connects bone to bone.

Lymph A fluid similar to plasma that circulates in the lymphatic system.

Lymphatic system A system of vessels and glands which collects strayed proteins leaked from blood vessels and cleanses the body of microbes and other foreign matter.

M

Mechanism of injury The force that causes an injury and the way it is applied to the body.

Medical help The treatment given by or under the supervision of a medical doctor.

Micro-organisms Germs which can cause illness.

Mouth-to-mouth ventilation Artificial respiration by blowing air into the mouth of a casualty.

Mucous membrane A thin, slick, transparent lining, covering tubes and internal organs such as the inner surface of the mouth, nose, eye, ear, intestine etc.

Musculoskeletal system All the bones, muscles and connecting tissues which allow movement.

Myocardial infarction Death of part of the cardiac (heart) muscle; heart attack.

N

Nerve Fibres that carry nerve impulses to and from the brain.

Nervous system The brain, spinal cord and nerves which control the body's activities.

Nitroglycerine A drug used to ease the workload on the heart; often carried as a pill or spray by people with angina.

O

Obstructed airway A blockage in the air passageway to the lungs.

Oxygen An odourless, colourless gas essential to life. (Symbol O_2).

P

Paralysis Inability to move, or loss of motor function in one or more parts of the body.

Physiology The study of the functions of the body.

Plasma A pale yellow fluid containing proteins, i.e. blood after the cells have been removed.

Pleural membrane A slick membrane covering the outside surface of the lungs and the inside surface of the chest cavity (thorax).

Pneumonia Inflammation of the lungs.

Pnuemothorax An accumulation of air in the pleural space. Normally the pleural space contains a negative pressure, or vacuum; the air mass (instead of a vacuum) collapses the lung under it.

Primary survey Assessing the casualty for life-threatening injuries and giving appropriate first aid.

Pulmonary artery The major artery emerging from the right ventricle; carries deoxygenated blood to the lungs.

Pulse The rhythmic expansion and relaxation of the arteries caused by the contractile force of the heart; usually felt where the vessels cross a bone near the surface.

R

Radiate Spreading from a central point; the pain of a heart attack in the chest radiates to the left arm.

Red blood cells The most numerous type of blood cells, which carry oxygen.

Respiratory arrest Stopped breathing.

Retina The lining at the back of the eyeball which converts light rays into nerve impulses.

RICE R=rest; I=ice; C=compression; E=elevation. First aid for certain bone and joint injuries.

Rule of Nines A system of estimating the amout of skin surface damaged in a burn injury.

S

Scene survey The initial step of ESM where the first aider takes control, assesses any hazards and makes the area safe, finds out what has happened, identifies him- or herself as a first aider, gains consent from the casualty, calls for help from bystanders and begins to organize them to get help for the casualty.

Secondary survey Assessing the casualty for non-life-threatening injuries and then giving appropriate first aid.

Sign Objective evidence of a disease or injury.

Spontaneous pneumothorax Air in the pleural space which has leaked from a weakened area of a lung.

Sprain Supporting tissues about a joint (such as ligaments) are stretched, partly or completely torn (*see also* **strain**).

Sternum The breastbone.

Strain A stretched muscle (*see also* **sprain**).

Sucking chest wound A chest wound through which air is pulled into the chest cavity. It can cause a collapse of the lung beneath.

Superficial On the surface of the body, as opposed to deep.

Symptom An indication of illness or injury experienced by a casualty; cannot be detected by an observer without asking.

T

Tendon A tough cord of tissue that attaches muscles to bones and other tissues.

Tetanus A type of bacteria which invades wounds and cause severe muscle spasms.

Transient ischaemic attack (TIA) Temporary signs and symptoms of a stroke due to a lack of sufficient oxygen to the brain.

Trachea Tube for air, kept open with cartilage rings; located between the larynx and the bronchi.

Traction Gently but firmly pulling below a fracture to bring the limb into alignment.

Trauma Any physical or psychological injury.

Triage A system of assigning priorities for first aid and/or transportation for multiple casualties.

V

Vein A blood vessel carrying blood to the heart.

Ventilation Supplying air to the lungs.

Ventricles The muscular lower chambers of the heart which pump blod to the arteries.

Ventricular fibrillation A quivering action of the heart muscles so that little or no blood is pumped into the arteries.

Vital signs Signs that show the basic condition of the casualty: breaths per minute, heart rate, temperature and level of consciousness.

W

White blood cells Blood cells which are involved in immunity and control of infection.

INDEX

Note: *italicized* page numbers refer to illustrated material.

CONTACTS AND SAFETY ORGANIZATIONS

UNITED KINGDOM
THE BRITISH RED CROSS
UK Office
44 Moorfields
London EC2Y 9AL
tel: +44 (0) 870 170 700
fax: +44 (0) 20 7562-2000
www.redcross.org.uk/

ST JOHN'S AMBULANCE
Priory House
25 St John's Lane
Clerkenwell
London
EC1M 4PP
England
tel: +44 (0) 20 7251-3292
fax: +44 (0) 20 7251-3287
email: secretariat@orderofstjohn.org

ROYAL SOCIETY FOR THE PREVENTION OF ACCIDENTS (ROSPA)
Edgbaston Park
353 Bristol Road
Edgbaston
Birmingham B5 7ST
England
tel: +44 (121) 248 2129
fax: +44 (121) 248 2001
email: help@rospa.co.uk
www.rospa.com

SOUTH AFRICA
CHILD ACCIDENT PREVENTION FOUNDATION OF SOUTH AFRICA (CAPFSA)
PO Box 791
Rondebosch 7701
South Africa
tel: +27 (21) 685-5208
fax: +27 (21) 685 5331
email: capfsa@pgwc.gov.za
www.altonsa.co.za/childsafe

FRANCE
COMMISSION DE LA SÉCURITÉ DES CONSOMMATEURS
Cité Martignac
111 rue de Grenelle
75353 Paris 07 SP
France
tel: +33 (1) 43 19 56 53
fax: +33 (1) 43 19 57 00
www.securiteconso.org

AUSTRALIA & NEW ZEALAND
KIDSAFE CHILD ACCIDENT PREVENTION TRUST (CAPT)
PO Box 3515
Parramatta NSW 2124
tel: +61 (2) 9845 0890
fax: + 61 (2) 9845 0895
www.kidsafe.com.au
www.kidsafe.com.nz

KIDSAFE ACCIDENT PREVENTION FOUNDATION
50 Kidsafe House
50 Bramston Terrace
Herston QLD 4029
Australia
tel: +61 (617) 3854 1829
fax: +61 (617) 3252 7900
email: qld@kidsafe.org.au
www.kidsafe.org.au

PHOTO CREDITS

Copyright rests with the following photographers and/or their agents as listed below. Key to locations: t = top; c = centre; b = bottom; l = left; r = right.

Anipix (Jan Castrium) = A/JA. **British Red Cross** = BRC. **Christel Clear** = CCl. **Colin Monteath** (Hedgehoghouse.com) = CM/H. **Images of Africa** = IoA (Shaen Adey = SA; Nancy Gardiner = NG; Anthony Johnson = AJ; Jacques Marais = JM; Ryno Reyneke = RR; Dorotheé van der Osten = DvO). **Photo Access** = PA. **Science Photo Library** = SPL (Dr M.A. Ansary = DrA; Connor Caffrey = CC; Mark Clarke = MC; Michael Donne = MD; John Greim = JG; Richard Hutchings = RH; Dr P.Marazzi = DrM; Chris Priest = CP; Mark Thomas = MT). **Warren Photographic** (Jane Burton) = WP/JB.

11		IoA/RR	80		IoA/DvO	127		SPL/CP & MC
25		BRC	93	tr	SPL/DrM	133		PA
26		BRC		bl	SPL/RH	135		SPL/CP
27		BRC	94	tl	SPL/DrA	143	tr	PA
29		BRC		tr	SPL	151	bl	IoA
30		BRC		bl	SPL/MC		br	IoA/NG
32		BRC	95	tl	SPL/DrM	154		IoA
35	bl	BRC	100	br	A/JA	155		CCl
36	2 x br	BRC	104		WP/JB	159		IoA
39	t	BRC	107		IoA/JM	160	bl	IoA/JM
41		BRC	118		CM/H	161	tr	IoA/JM
43	tr	SPL/MT	119		IoA/JM	162	bl	IoA/AJ
62		PA	124		SPL/JG		br	IoA/SA
72		PA	125		SPL/CC			
75		IoA/JM	126		SPL/MD			

ACKNOWLEDGEMENTS

The publisher would like to thank everyone who participated so enthusiastically in the photo shoots, in particular: Heather Baker, Helaine Beukes, Elroy Cameron, Lloyd Christopher, Marjory Dobell, Jarryd and Justin Florentino, Carla and Robyn Kellermann, Lee Maneveldt of St John's Ambulance for the loan of first aid kits, Dr Cleeve Robertson, Victor Tiludi, P. J. van Tonder, J.A. van Tonder, D. A. Winter, Kat Ziegenhagen, Ron van Til for providing the DIY props.

PERSONAL EMERGENCY RECORD

Ambulance/emergency service...

Hospital ....

Doctor ....

Paediatrician ....

Dentist ....

Pharmacy ....

Fire brigade ....

Police ....

Poison centre ....

Relative ....

Friend ....

Neighbour ....

School ....

Dad Work ....

Mom Work ....

Vet ....

Electricity ....

Gas ....

Water ....

Insurance company ....